Financing
Long-Term
Care

THE CRUCIAL DEBATE

William Laing

B O O K S

© 1993 William Laing
Published by Age Concern England
1268 London Road
London SW16 4ER

Editor Caroline Hartnell
Production Marion Peat
Design and typesetting Eugenie Dodd
Copy preparation Vinnette Marshall
Printed in Great Britain by Hartnolls Ltd, Cornwall

A catalogue record for this book is available
from the British Library.

ISBN 0–86242–123–3

CONTENTS

ABOUT THE AUTHOR

After graduating from the London School of Economics, William Laing joined the Association of the British Pharmaceutical Industry (ABPI) in 1967 as an economist. Subsequently he transferred to the ABPI-sponsored Office of Health Economics (OHE) where he was appointed Deputy Director in 1971. During his time at the OHE he researched and wrote a number of occasional papers in the OHE's series on the economic and social aspects of health.

In 1976 William Laing left the OHE to set up a company which subsequently specialised in publications, conferences and consultancy in the growing independent health care sector. He now edits two widely respected annual publications, *Laing's Review of Private Healthcare*, which is acknowledged as the authoritative annual reference source on the activities of the independent sector, and *Care of Elderly People*, a comprehensive review of structure and trends in the long-term care industry. He has a special interest in the funding of long-term care for elderly people and is the joint author of *The Challenges of Ageing*, published by the ABPI in 1991 as part of the *Agenda for Health* series. He is also the author of *Empowering the Elderly: Direct consumer funding of care services*, published by the Institute of Economic Affairs Health and Welfare Unit in 1991, in which he argues for state funding for care services to be channelled to service users themselves.

1 Introduction

The United Kingdom, like other developed countries, needs to finance the rapidly growing demand for long-term care for elderly people over the coming decades. The underlying demographic causes are well known. This century has already witnessed a large increase in the number of very old people, who have the highest propensity to use care services. By 1992 about 1.5 per cent of GDP was being spent on long-term care services for elderly people, in addition to a very large amount of care provided by unpaid carers which does not enter into the national accounts. Looking further ahead into the next century, the ageing of the baby boom generation of 1950–65 combined with falling mortality rates will lead to a further inexorable rise in expenditure. The results of the 1991 census are now available, and the latest, 1991-based, principal population projection by the Government Actuary envisages a much more rapid expansion in the number of very old people than had previously been calculated. Using these new data, and assuming that age-specific use rates for long-term care services remain constant at their present levels, national expenditure on such services can be projected to rise to a peak of 3.5 per cent of GDP by the middle of the twenty-first century, by which time there would be well over 1 million people living in residential or nursing homes. Though the magnitude of the sums that will be spent may be debated, the fact that a major shift of resources into long-term care is required is not in doubt.

The fundamental question addressed in this book is whether there exists at present an equitable, efficient and affordable system for financing increasing volumes of long-term care now and in the decades to come and, if not, what public policy options exist for creating such a system.

This raises a broader set of issues than those addressed by Sir Roy Griffiths in his inquiry into community care (HMSO, 1988a) and by the government in its subsequent policy decisions, culminating in the transfer of most state finance for long-term care services to local authorities from April 1993. The broader issues discussed in this book include the merits of a social insurance model for state funding of long-term care, in place of the present mainly means-tested system, and, more generally, the merits of private versus public insurance in financing long-term care. Though Sir Roy Griffiths' report did briefly refer to private sources of long-term care funding, such as home equity release and employer-funded schemes, the government remit he was following for reforming community care was essentially restricted to finding new ways of administering the existing, predominantly means-tested, system of state funding. Moreover, in the period of policy implementation that followed the Griffiths report, there has been little if any debate on the wider policy issues or options relating to the totality of private and public funding of long-term care now and in the twenty-first century.

▪ The rest of the book

Chapters 2–6 provide background information on long-term care funding in the United Kingdom, which will be useful in understanding the public policy issues and options discussed in Chapter 7.

Chapter 2 looks briefly at the history of long-term care financing. It identifies the crucial distinction that was drawn in 1948 between the National Health Service, financed on a universal basis and available to all irrespective of means, and long-term care, which was made largely subject to a means test under the National Assistance Act. It further concludes that financing arrangements for long-term care, whether in the public, private or voluntary sectors, have lagged decades behind financing arrangements for other important economic needs, for example health care, pensions and house purchase.

The rapid growth of Income Support as a source of state funding in the 1980s and early 1990s is highlighted and the principal financial features of the community care reforms incorporated in the 1990 NHS and Community Care Act are described. Following implementation in April 1993, the Act has transferred responsibility for state funding for people entering independent sector residential and nursing homes from the open-ended Income Support account, with no needs assessment, to cash-limited local authority budgets, with needs assessment. It is concluded that state funding for the long-term care of elderly people will almost certainly grow less rapidly in the remainder of the 1990s than in the previous decade.

Chapter 3 describes the main features of long-term care financing in the UK from both state and personal sources, and gives details of the current means-testing regime. It estimates annual spending on the long-term care of elderly people at £9.1 billion (annualised at April 1992). Of this total, 73 per cent (£6.6 billion) was spent on long-term care in NHS or care home settings and the remaining £2.5 billion on long-term care for people living in their own homes. Analysed by source of funds, 70 per cent (£6.3 billion) was spent by the state while the remaining 30 per cent (£2.8 billion) came from personal income and wealth.

It is expected that personal expenditure will increase its share of total spending, in the short term because the local authority-operated means test excludes more people from state funding than did the old Income Support means test, as explained on pages 41–44, and in the long term because the higher rates of property ownership (which usually renders people ineligible for state funding for residential or nursing home care) will filter through to the very old population at risk of needing care services.

The phenomenon of 'informal selectivism' for local authority services for people living in their own homes is identified. This refers to the tendency of local authorities to concentrate their domiciliary care resources on people who live alone and do not have a relative or friend to care for them, while people who already have the support of a heavily involved carer may typically be left to cope by themselves. Informal means-testing selects against certain classes of carer rather than against certain recipients of care, the criterion for selection being the availability of care provided by unpaid carers rather than the availability of income or assets. In all other respects, however, the principle of 'informal selectivism' on which local authority domiciliary services are usually based very closely parallels the financial selectivism of local authority-funded residential and nursing home care, and raises precisely the same equity issues as the more familiar concept of financial selectivism.

Using a method of calculation similar to that used by the Family Policy Studies Centre, the total 'value' of care provided by unpaid carers for elderly people is calculated at £32.5 billion in 1992, dwarfing the amount spent on formal care services. This estimate is derived by valuing each hour of unpaid care at £7, based on local authority costs.

It is estimated that about £1 billion in Attendance Allowance and Disability Living Allowance was paid to elderly people living in private households in 1992/93 but only about half that amount was spent on aids and adaptations or care services.

Chapter 3 also identifies the unresolved issues in long-term funding. These include the responsibility of the NHS for paying for long-term nursing care, the appropriateness of means-testing, the merits of a budget-capped system of state funding with no clearly stated entitlements, concerns over empowerment of consumers, and the broad issue of the role of private versus public financing.

Chapter 4 deals with personal payment for long-term care. It is predicted that the proportion of long-term care spending funded from personal sources (whether income, assets, family contributions or specially designed long-term care financial products) will increase in the future. In the short term it will increase because of the more stringent means-testing regime applied by local authorities since April 1993. In the longer term it will increase as high rates of owner occupation filter through to the very elderly population most at risk of needing care services. This trend will continue as long as property ownership disqualifies individuals from means-tested state benefits for residential or nursing home care.

Private long-term care funding products were first introduced on to the UK market in 1991. Five types of product are described, which can be classified into two broad groups. The first group consists of prefunded plans such as long-term care insurance, where the individual pays for a number of years in advance and does not know whether he or she will need to claim. The second group consists of immediate care products such as annuities or equity release, where the individual needs to finance care services immediately and typically pays out of house equity. Sales for both of these groups have been slow since they were launched in 1991. The main barriers to sales are perceived to be price and lack of awareness of the need to make provision.

Though increasing numbers of elderly people can finance a significant duration of care in a residential or nursing home through liquidation of house equity and other assets, possibly linked with the purchase of immediate care products, only a minority of elderly people in the UK will be able to afford to pay for prefunded private financial products out of income for the foreseeable future. A similar conclusion has been reached by researchers in the USA.

All but one of the prefunded long-term care products introduced in the UK have used Activities of Daily Living (ADLs) as the trigger for benefits. The advantage of ADLs is that they are reasonably objective and transparent – that is, it is clearly evident how decisions about level of entitlement are reached. The disadvantage of ADLs is poor targeting, given the widely differing care needs of individuals with the same ADL profile. ADL-triggered insurance therefore has an in-built tendency towards cost inflation relative to state-funded long-term care programmes, which aim to tailor packages of care to meet the requirements of each individual.

Chapter 5 compares the UK system of financing long-term care with the systems adopted by selected OECD (Organisation for Economic Co-operation and Development) countries. These can be divided into five types along the continuum from universality (the social insurance principle) to selectivism (means-testing – the welfare principle):

1 Social insurance entitlement with no charges: no country meets this criterion.

2 Social insurance entitlement with flat-rate charges for long-term care outside people's own homes: Canada only.

3 Social insurance for care coupled with welfare benefits for the hotel costs of long-term care outside people's own homes: France and, in the future, Germany.

4 Income-tested welfare benefits for both care and hotel elements of long-term care outside people's own homes: Sweden.

5 Income- and asset-tested welfare benefits for both care and hotel elements of long-term care outside people's own homes: UK, United States, the Netherlands and, at present, Germany.

The UK state funding system is at the more severely means-tested end of the means-testing spectrum for long-term care outside people's own homes, but it is by no means atypical. For long-term care services for people living in their own homes the UK means-testing regime is squarely located in the European mainstream.

In no country does the private financial services sector yet play a significant role with financial products specifically designed to pay for long-term care services. Long-term care insurance is most highly developed in the United States. It currently accounts for only 1 per cent of nursing home revenues but 4 per cent of people aged 65 and over are insured.

Chapter 6 poses the question: how big is the demographic time bomb? Age-specific rates of usage of long-term care services are given and a method is described for projecting future spending on long-term care for elderly people – from 1.5 per cent of GDP in 1992 to a peak of 3.5 per cent of GDP in 2051. The longer-term the projection, the more uncertain it becomes. Medical technology is probably the most important wild card, and two opposing hypotheses are given on the impact medical technology may have on care costs. The 'optimistic' hypothesis is championed by Fries, who maintains that a process of compression of morbidity is taking place, in which the onset of chronic ill-health is being delayed and the period of dependency before death is being compressed. The opposing 'pessimistic' theory, put forward by Kramer and Gruenberg, holds that the recent fall in mortality rates among elderly people, observed in all Western countries, has not been accompanied by a similar decline in morbidity rates, and that the ratio of disability-free to total life expectancy is declining. The conclusion drawn is that the evidence one way or the other is insufficiently strong to alter the way in which we should plan the funding of long-term care in future years.

The other major uncertainty in future years is the extent to which people remain willing and able to provide unpaid care for elderly relatives. Divorce, changes in women's working patterns and geographical dispersal of families have all been cited as manifestations of a break-up of traditional family structures which may threaten the bedrock of such care. The conclusion drawn, however, is that there is as yet little evidence to support some of the more alarmist predictions about the diminishing availability of care provided by unpaid carers.

The rate of inflation in the unit cost of care is flagged as a further factor which might in theory cause long-term care costs to escalate out of control. More stringent regulation, rising expectations and the development of private long-term care insurance may all have an inflationary effect. Countervailing deflationary influences include state funding constraints and more efficient delivery of care services. Again, it is concluded that there is little to support the more alarmist predictions.

In the light of the analysis of previous chapters, Chapter 7 presents the fundamental policy issues and options that need to be addressed. A small number of 'candidate' policy ideas are selected as being worthy of attention in the national debate which is believed to be long overdue on the financing of long-term care services for elderly people.

The main policy issues are stated as follows:

1   Is long-term care a risk that the state should cover?

2   Is there a case for non-means-tested social insurance for long-term care?

3   Should the government encourage private financial provision for care in old age, and, if so, how?

4   Is the balance right between funding of services and income supplementation?

5   How should the government promote efficiency and individual choice in long-term care services?

All these questions relate to the structure of the financing system, which is the central concern of this book. The question of the adequacy of public sector long-term care budgets is not addressed here.

Is long-term care a risk that the state should cover?

The major gap which is identified in the welfare state safety net is not so much services for elderly people themselves as support and compensation for carers, whose massive contribution of unpaid care dwarfs the amount of paid long-term care services.

Carers may suffer severe financial and other burdens, be denied significant protection from the state, and have no realistic private insurance alternative. Of all the gaps in the welfare state's arrangements for covering long-term care risks, therefore, this appears to merit the most urgent review on equity grounds. On public expenditure grounds, too, there *may* be a case for increased financial support for carers, if such support can be shown to have the effect of preventing people withdrawing from the provision of unpaid care, with the catastrophic effects that would have on local authority care budgets.

Is there a case for non-means-tested social insurance?

The overriding issue here is the public expenditure cost. If a non-means-tested entitlement to state funding of long-term care services were introduced in the UK, the effect might be to increase the proportion of long-term care funded by the state from the present 70 per cent to 90 per cent, at a public expenditure cost of £1.8 billion in 1992, or 0.3 per cent of GDP. By the year 2051, because of the ageing population, the additional cost of non-means-tested social insurance for long-term care can be projected to reach 0.7 per cent of GDP.

There are broadly three equity arguments in favour of non-means-tested state funding. The first concerns inter-generational equity. People who find that the state will pay for little if any of their long-term care costs in old age may complain that they have been sold a false prospectus by the state. The second concerns intra-generational equity. Thrifty individuals may get no state long-term care benefits until they have exhausted their resources while the spendthrift, having saved nothing, gets immediate financial assistance from the state under the means-testing system. The third broad argument in favour of non-means-tested social insurance for long-term care is that the state ought at least to pay for all *health* care irrespective of means, the definition of health to include all nursing care, which is now more frequently provided on a means-tested basis in independent nursing homes than free in NHS long-stay facilities.

The final element of the equity argument relates to the effect of any move away from means-testing on the distribution of income and wealth. One effect would be to redistribute resources in favour of frail elderly people in need of long-term care. But the principal effect, in practice, would be to conserve assets for elderly people to pass on at death. This would be welcomed by those who wish to see wealth, largely in the form of house equity, cascading down generations. But it has to be asked whether it is sensible to cut other public sector spending or raise new taxes to support a programme whose principal effect is to enlarge the pool of often well-off people receiving inheritances on the death of their parents.

In summary, there are elements of inequity in the existing system of state funding of long-term care, but the case for the state to take on a major new social insurance programme for the financing of long-term care in order to resolve them is by no means clear-cut. If, on balance, it is believed that there is merit in reducing the degree of means-testing for long-term care, the two most practical options open to the state are, first, minor modifications of the means-testing regime and, second, introduction of a partial social insurance scheme.

Minor modifications of the means-testing regime might aim to relieve its most severe effects. For example, the assets disregard limit of £8,000, beyond which individuals are ineligible for state support to enter residential or nursing home care, might be raised and the tariff income rule might be modified. Relaxation of these rules would particularly help people with a moderate level of assets who wish to enter a care home where the charges are higher than the local authority is willing to cover, but who are worried that the limited disregard leaves them with insufficient resources over and above state benefits to assure their continued ability to meet the extra charges until death. Minor modifications like this would go some way towards addressing the intra-generational equity issue, but the other equity issues raised by means-testing would remain unresolved.

The most rational policy option is the *partial* social insurance model which is used in France and is about to be adopted in Germany. This stands out clearly as a means of resolving many of the equity issues and removing the remaining perverse incentives in the UK state funding system. It would, however, be expensive in public expenditure terms, though less expensive than a fully comprehensive social insurance scheme.

A partial social insurance scheme would make long-term *care* in a residential or nursing home a non-means-tested state benefit, subject only to assessment of need, but would continue the present severe means-testing regime for the *hotel* element of care. At its most rational, the non-means-tested care entitlement would extend to 'social' as well as 'nursing' care in order to avoid the arbitrary distinctions that are currently made between the two, in the UK and elsewhere.

One way of mitigating the additional public expenditure cost would be to introduce hotel charges for NHS long-stay hospital beds. Presented as part of a package of reforms offering extended social insurance cover for long-term care, any political objections to charging for NHS services would carry much less weight.

A partial social insurance scheme along the lines described would encourage sales of private financial products for long-term care, provided the social insurance benefit could be used as a 'voucher' and supplemented from private resources.

Should the government encourage private funding mechanisms?

The scope for the private sector to take over the burden of long-term care funding from the public sector is limited. The evidence from the UK and other countries is that prefunded private financial products which offer comprehensive long-term care cover are too expensive to envisage voluntary purchase replacing a substantial proportion of state funding in the foreseeable future. The main justification for encouraging private sector initiatives is that they increase choice and may improve the quality of life and peace of mind of the minority who can afford them.

It is concluded that the case for tax concessions to encourage private funding vehicles for long-term care is weak, except possibly for

certain highly targeted products. Moreover, most insurance companies involved in developing and marketing financial products for
funding long-term care would broadly accept that, subject to certain
modifications, the present tax environment does not unduly hinder
the development of such products.

There is, however, a strong case for measures to resolve existing
anomalies in the tax and regulatory treatment of long-term care funding products and a number of specific recommendations are made.

Apart from modifying the tax regime, the government might also
consider introducing limited exemptions from the normal means-
testing regime in order to stimulate the development of private long-
term care funding products designed to complement state benefits. At
present there is little scope for complementary products because, for
residential and nursing home care, any benefit from a private financial
product would reduce state benefits pound for pound.

An example of such an initiative in the United States, the Connecticut Health Partnership, is described. A hypothetical product
designed for the British market, a single-premium delayed annuity, is
also described.

There are, however, equity objections to all such initiatives designed specifically to stimulate the private financial services sector.
Why, it may be asked, should individuals who happen to have purchased approved long-term care financing products be exempted from
ordinary means tests while others are not?

Balance between funding of services and income supplementation

Income supplementation is most appropriate where large numbers of
individuals receive fairly small sums, where the objective of the benefit is as much compensation as service provision, and where the range
of relevant service provision may be too wide to define easily.

There is a strong case for carers – and particularly co-resident,
long-term carers, who are among those most disadvantaged by the
existing arrangements for funding long-term care – to receive any
additional state help through the social security system where
defined rules of entitlement prevent the inequitable prioritisation that

may take place within third-party state funding agencies such as local authorities.

Promotion of individual choice in long-term care

Fears about the excessive discretionary powers of local authority budget-holders were allayed by the government decision to enshrine state-funded individuals' right to choice of care home in statutory guidance. There is no such guidance, however, for services for people living in their own homes, where local and health authorities will continue to exercise purchasing discretion on behalf of their clients.

Empowerment of elderly consumers of state-funded care services might be achieved by local authorities making cash available to service users themselves, to spend on care services of their own choice with the aid, if they wish, of care service 'brokers'. Brokers should be accountable to service users, not to local authorities. Those users who do not want to exercise control in any way would be free to leave their cash allocation with the local authority social services department to spend on their behalf.

The proposed scheme would, it is argued, enhance choice and stimulate innovation in the delivery of care services, as suppliers responded to the perceived needs of elderly people themselves. It would also be wholly consistent with 'partial social insurance', identified above as the most promising policy option for resolving inequities and removing the remaining perverse incentives from the present system of state financing.

▪ Definitions of key terms

Long-term care is defined to embrace all forms of continuing personal or nursing care and associated domestic services for people who are unable to look after themselves without some degree of support, whether provided in their own homes, at a day centre, or in an NHS or care home setting. Long-term care is essentially for people who are not going to get better. It excludes 'acute' medical care, aimed at curing or alleviating particular medical conditions. Though the distinction between 'long-term' and 'acute' may be conceptually fuzzy, in practice it is usually fairly clear.

Long-term care for people living in their own homes includes such services as alarm systems, meals on wheels, home helps/home care workers and home nurses – in addition to the more flexible and imaginative packages of care that are now emerging to support people in their own homes. It includes 'close care', 'housing with care' and other variants on very sheltered housing, in which people move to a location where centralised care is available, but in an environment which enables them to retain a substantial degree of independence. It also covers care provided in day centres and day hospitals.

Long-term care in NHS or care home settings includes private, voluntary and local authority residential homes, private and voluntary nursing homes and NHS long-stay hospitals for elderly and elderly mentally ill people. Residential and nursing homes are sometimes referred to collectively as 'care homes'. Private and voluntary care homes may be referred to as 'independent' care homes.

2 History of long-term care financing in the UK

There is always a risk, especially when writing at the invitation of an organisation which represents a particular section of the community, of falling into the trap of special pleading. Every effort has been made to avoid tendentiousness. Nevertheless, it is difficult to escape the conclusion that public and private arrangements for financing long-term care have lagged decades behind financing arrangements for other important economic needs, for example health care, pensions and house purchase. This is not something which is unique to the United Kingdom. Other industrialised countries have been similarly slow to develop financing arrangements to ensure ready access to a comprehensive range of good quality care services if and when they are needed. Presumably, society and the individuals within society have only been willing to consider devoting substantial resources to assuring comprehensive long-term care services in frail and dependent old age when an advanced stage of economic development has been reached and when other, higher priorities such as medical care, education, sickness and unemployment benefits and pensions have been adequately catered for.

▪ History of public sector financing

Central government involvement in long-term care financing in Britain grew out of the system for poor relief. Its origins can be traced back to the Elizabethan Poor Relief Act of 1601, under which poor houses were gradually developed to house paupers of all kinds – young, old, sick, infirm, mentally handicapped and mentally ill – in a single custodial institution run by the parish. They could hardly be described as 'caring' institutions, though eventually, several centuries later, residential care services did emerge from their successors, the Victorian workhouses, constructed following the Poor Law Amendment Act of 1834.

During the nineteenth and early twentieth centuries, with economic growth, expanding education services and the beginnings of social insurance, there was a gradual reduction in the number of younger and able-bodied people forced to seek indoor (workhouse) relief. Workhouses were left with a residual population of old and infirm residents, which in turn brought about a change in attitude from the harsh authoritarianism of the nineteenth century to the more benign approach of the mid-twentieth century. Some workhouses were reclassified as local authority-run hospitals. Nevertheless, when the National Assistance Act was passed in 1948, public funding of long-term care for elderly people was still focused on poor relief in old poor law institutions.

Such improvements as there were in the conditions of dependent elderly people owed more to spin-offs from developments in other areas of social security than to policies aimed specifically at the dependent elderly client group. The primary domestic preoccupation of government during the early part of the twentieth century was with establishing health and unemployment insurance and basic pensions. These new benefits enabled more elderly people to maintain their independence, or get support from their families. But the notion of directly addressing the need for a financial framework to assure long-term care services for dependent people had not yet emerged on the policy agenda.

Moreover, when the institutions of the welfare state were being created immediately after the Second World War, dependent elderly and infirm people continued to be treated essentially as a residual category under the new order. The principle of social insurance, whereby eligible individuals became entitled to benefits regardless of income or assets, was applied to health, education, sickness benefits, unemployment benefits and pensions. State provision for the long-term care of elderly people who were sick or infirm was the responsibility of the

NHS, while care of the frail and old rested with local government. The former was free, the latter means-tested.

A fundamental distinction between acute health care, as a universally available state benefit, and long-term care for elderly people, as a benefit which is (usually) selectively available according to means, was thus drawn at the inception of the welfare state in Britain. In nearly all other developed countries, though their institutions differ, the same distinction has broadly been made and continues to apply today. Among the countries whose funding systems are described in Chapter 5, only Canada provides access to long-term care outside people's own homes as a social insurance benefit available to all insured people irrespective of means. All other countries make state funding of long-term care outside people's own homes depend on means-testing to a greater or lesser extent, with the UK located towards the more rigorous and selective end of the means-testing range.

▪ History of voluntary sector financing

Historically, the voluntary sector has given the needs of dependent elderly people a similarly low priority. Though some outdoor (outside the workhouse) relief for elderly people was financed by voluntary bodies in the nineteenth century, when only indoor relief was available from the state, the main thrust of voluntary action in nineteenth-century Britain was in acute health care rather than the long-term care of elderly people. The voluntary hospitals which flourished in the nineteenth century were places of research and teaching in medical care, which performed those functions with the aid of a rapid throughput of acutely sick patients. They could not afford to finance long-term care.

Those voluntary establishments which were developed to cater for long-term care were often run by religious institutions or orders, following a much older tradition which had been interrupted in the sixteenth century by the dissolution of the monasteries in Britain. Otherwise, voluntary establishments were set up by employers' organisations to cater for particular occupational groups. To a limited extent, some charities also addressed the care needs of elderly people through the provision of housing.

The friendly societies which flourished for working and lower middle class people in the nineteenth and early twentieth centuries were, like the state itself, more concerned with sickness and unemployment benefits, payment for medical care and basic pensions. There was no scope for the 'luxury' of enhanced benefits to pay for additional care services for dependent elderly people.

▪ History of private sector financing

In common with the public and voluntary sectors, private sector arrangements for financing the long-term care of dependent elderly people have historically been slow to develop. Informal family support is supposed to have been the mainstay of care for elderly people in Victorian and Edwardian Britain, with large families producing at least one unmarried daughter to look after ageing parents. But the further down the social scale, the more likely this is to have been a myth (Thompson, 1986; Gordon, 1988).

Of all of the private sector institutions which developed in the early twentieth century, occupational pension schemes were those with the greatest potential scope for financing long-term care in old age. The state had always led the way in occupational pension provision in Britain, with its superannuation fund for civil servants. It was in the 1930s that private enterprise began to make an important contribution to the development of retirement benefits. According to Trebilcock (1985) the initial impulse came from the United States, where large company pension schemes were already well established, with benefits often being provided under a group contract issued to the employer by an insurance company. Some schemes were imported into Britain for employees of British subsidiaries of American parent companies, and British insurers soon entered this market themselves. Schemes provided pensions, death benefits and in some cases a disability income and widow's pension. The most generous, therefore, would have helped to pay for some care services. But although they went close, they did not set out specifically to finance long-term care for elderly former employees.

More recently, the postwar growth of owner occupation has created the conditions for potentially massive private funding of long-term care services for people living in their own homes by borrowing money against the value of their property, but to date equity release has been slow to develop and it is probable that few of those elderly people who have purchased such plans have used substantial amounts of the additional income to fund care services.

In contrast, home equity is the principal source of private funding for long-term care in residential or nursing homes – either directly, following the sale of a formerly owner-occupied house, or indirectly, where family members provide funding in anticipation of being the beneficiaries of the estate on the elderly person's death. It is only in the last two years, however, that the private financial services sector has introduced products designed specifically to translate house equity (or capital from other sources) into revenue streams to pay for residential and nursing home care.

It is also only in the last two years that prefunded financial products such as long-term care insurance and modified personal pension schemes specifically designed to finance long-term care have been introduced in Britain. In most other OECD countries, too, private funding products are still at an early stage of development. Only in the United States has long-term care insurance been established for a number of years, with 4 per cent of people aged 65 and over insured.

In summary, therefore, public, voluntary and private institutions have all been slow to respond to the challenge of financing long-term care services for elderly people, in other countries as well as in Britain. In the great movements and reforms of the past, elderly people needing long-term care have typically been treated as a residual category, for whom specific financial arrangements have been the exception rather than the rule. It is only very recently that the need for comprehensive financing arrangements specifically for dependent elderly people has started to be addressed seriously. Elderly people and their families currently make use of a patchwork of state and private funding, crucially supported by care provided by unpaid carers. The aim of this book is to ask whether this patchwork is adequate to take the UK into the next century.

■ From Income Support to the community care reforms

The first 30 years of the postwar welfare state in the UK witnessed a broad expansion of state-financed long-term care services for elderly people, almost exclusively provided in public sector facilities. But under the budget-capped system for allocating public funds there were severe supply constraints. Access to local authority Part III accommodation for elderly people was rationed, and 'bed blocking' was a major problem for NHS hospital wards unable to discharge elderly patients to alternative care.

The stresses in the system became overwhelming when, following Britain's monetary crisis in 1976, capital for the expansion of Part III accommodation ceased to be available. In the years which followed, voluntary organisations also found their income from cash-strapped local authorities rapidly dwindling. In 1974 local authorities paid for about 60 per cent of voluntary sector residential home places in England. By 1983 this figure had dropped to 34 per cent. The voluntary organisations started to look for an alternative source of money and found it in the social security system. Responding to pressure orchestrated and articulated by voluntary organisations, local social security offices started to pay Supplementary Benefit to people unable to afford their own fees and for whom local authorities were unwilling to foot the bill. Initially there was no national policy governing what were known as board and lodging allowances, but the practice became so widespread that policy was formalised in 1983 when, in effect, the government set up a voucher system for public funding of private and voluntary care homes. The rules that were introduced allowed anyone with less than £3,000 in capital and who qualified on income grounds to apply as of right for Supplementary Benefit to pay for admission to a residential or nursing home of their choice, provided it was a private or voluntary home. Benefit was not available to pay for local authority residential homes, nor, of course, could it be claimed to pay for NHS long-stay hospitals, since the NHS cannot charge for in-patient care of NHS patients. No assessment of need for residential or nursing home care was required. In its essentials, this new source of public funding remained in place until April 1993, though the initially generous locally determined weekly fee limits were subsequently replaced by much lower national limits, annually reviewed, while the £3,000 capital limit was subsequently raised to £8,000.

Figure 1 Places in nursing and residential homes and NHS long-stay hospitals for elderly, chronically ill and physically disabled people by sector, England, March 1967–92[a]

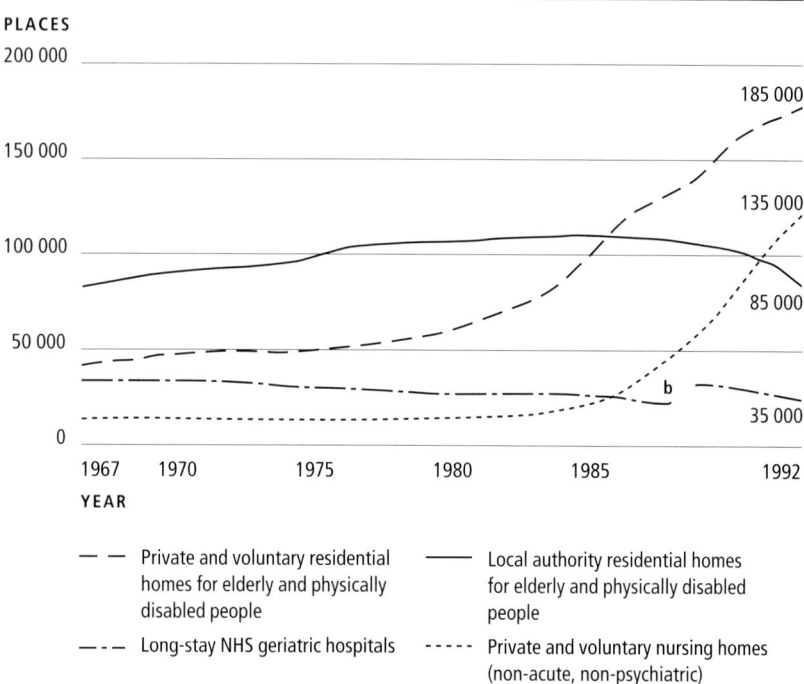

PLACES

Private and voluntary residential homes for elderly and physically disabled people

Local authority residential homes for elderly and physically disabled people

Long-stay NHS geriatric hospitals

Private and voluntary nursing homes (non-acute, non-psychiatric)

Notes: [a] Figures for places have always included younger physically disabled people.

[b] Discontinuity due to changes in definition. After 1988, separate figures for acute/rehabilitation geriatric beds and long-stay geriatric beds are no longer available. Long-stay beds have therefore been estimated since 1988 on the assumption that the number of acute/rehabilitation geriatric beds in England has remained constant and all the decline in the number of geriatric beds is attributable to the loss of long-stay beds.

Source: Laing and Buisson, 1993a.

Though voluntary organisations led the campaign for the new source of public funding, the principal beneficiaries in a business sense have been private providers of care homes. There is no doubt that the availability of Supplementary Benefit (renamed Income Support with the 1988 social security changes) fuelled the rapid expansion of private residential homes. It also fuelled the expansion of private nursing homes, though somewhat later (see Figure 1).

In no other area has public sector spending escalated so dramatically over the past decade as in Income Support funding of long-term care in residential and nursing homes (see *Table 1*).

Table 1 Income Support recipients in private and voluntary residential and nursing homes (all client types), Great Britain

YEAR	Numbers	Average payment [a] £ per week	Annualised expenditure £ million
December 1979	11 000	18	10
December 1980	13 000	27	18
December 1981	13 000	34	23
December 1982	16 000	47	39
December 1983	26 000	77	104
December 1984	42 000	92	200
December 1985	70 000	96	348
February 1986	90 000	98	459
May 1987	117 000	110	671
November 1987	130 100	114	772
May 1988	147 000	115	878
November 1988	155 000	119	958
May 1990	189 000	129	1 270
May 1991	231 000 [b]	156	1 870 [c]
November 1991	253 200 [d]	–	2 400 [d]
1992 estimate	–	–	2 530 [c]

Notes: [a] Income Support payments are net of other social security benefits and do not therefore give an accurate picture of total charges met from all social security sources.

[b] Hansard 21 October 1991, Vol 196 c 431 Written Answers.

[c] Hansard 17 November 1992, Vol 214 c 191 Written Answers.

[d] Hansard 15 May 1992, Vol 207 c 224–5 Written Answers.

Source: Department of Social Security.

The new source of funding had a number of important effects, some to the advantage of dependent elderly people, some to their disadvantage.

- Income Support is not cash-limited and overall state funding of care services for elderly people almost certainly grew faster than it would otherwise have done in the 1980s, even allowing for the fact that the NHS shed some of its long-stay hospital provision.

- Income Support funding enhanced consumer choice for elderly people in receipt of state-funded care, though the choice was crucially restricted to care home settings and to those parts of the country where there was a reasonable availability of care homes at or around national Income Support rates.

- The ready availability of Income Support funding for residential and nursing home care, but not for services for people living in their own homes, had the perverse effect of encouraging care in care home rather than home settings, totally at odds with espoused official policy objectives.

- Income Support funding created perverse incentives for both NHS and local authorities to shift part of the cost of their care services away from their own (cash-limited) budgets. Though the government created rules to prevent them from organising the transfer of particular residents to private or voluntary care homes, where they could receive Income Support, both health and local authorities did effectively shift the financial burden to Income Support by the expedient of rationing their own provision.

- The shift in provision out of NHS long-stay hospitals and into independent care homes meant a corresponding shift away from non-means-tested state financing and towards means-tested state financing, with the larger element of expenditure from personal sources which that involves. In 1970, 28 per cent of all elderly people receiving long-term care outside their own homes received 'free' NHS care. By 1992 this figure had fallen to 12 per cent.

The 250-fold increase in Income Support spending between 1979 and 1992 has been adduced as evidence that the ready availability of Income Support led to public spending escalating out of control.

Taken out of context, however, these statistics are misleading. The 'escalation' of Income Support took place at a time when demographic pressures were creating more demand while public sector provision was static or declining. *Figure 2* gives a more balanced illustration of the impact of Income Support. This uses a methodology originally developed by Laing and Buisson and subsequently used by the Firth Committee (DHSS, 1987) to estimate an index of demand for all types of long-term care in NHS and care home settings, after adjusting for changes in the age structure of the population.

Figure 2 Age-standardised index of supply: Private, voluntary, local authority and NHS long-stay places for elderly people in England combined (March 1981 = 100)

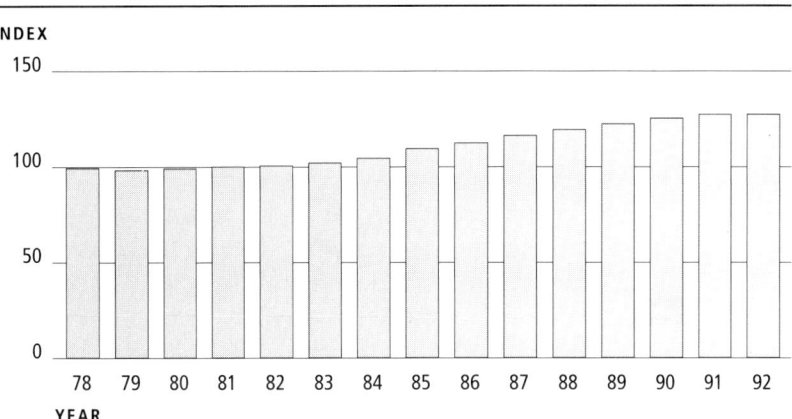

INDEX

YEAR

Notes: ᵃ Ratio of observed to expected places, the latter being the number that would have been observed in a given year if England 1981 age-specific rates of occupation of residential homes (grossed up to places of all types for long-term care of elderly people outside their own homes) are applied to the population in that year.

Source: Laing and Buisson, 1993a.

Figure 2 shows clearly that the emergence of readily available board and lodging allowances (subsequently Income Support) was followed by a substantial – but not unmanageable – increase in the number of people receiving some form of long-term care outside their own homes. By 1992 an estimated 27 per cent more elderly people were in long-term care establishments than would have been the case if age-specific rates had remained unchanged from a base year of 1981.

Even at this increased level, however, the UK has a lower rate of institutionalisation than most OECD countries (Doty, 1988).

The surge in demand which started in the early 1980s has been interpreted as evidence for elderly people being drawn unnecessarily into care homes. But an equally valid interpretation is that local authorities controlled admission into Part III residential homes so rigorously during the 1970s that any relaxation of admission criteria would have led to an increase in admissions.

Such hard evidence as there is seems to support the latter interpretation. Professor Bradshaw's team at the University of York, in work carried out for the DHSS, found that only 7 per cent of a sample of elderly people admitted to residential homes on Supplementary Benefit were inappropriately admitted on ordinary local authority criteria, given the alternative services then available (Bradshaw and Gibbs, 1988). If additional services such as sheltered housing or day care had been available it was judged that 10 per cent would not have needed to be admitted to a care home, and if full-time night sitting services had been available, 17 per cent of residents could have avoided admission. At this level of dependency, however, care in people's own homes may well be a more expensive option than care in a care home.

Such quantitative data as exist thus indicate that the ready availability of Income Support 'vouchers' had a relatively modest effect on the numbers of people entering care homes. (Against this some commentators have argued that Bradshaw looked only at admissions and that a much higher proportion of residents may become fit to return home but stay unnecessarily in care homes because care home owners have a strong financial incentive not to discharge them. Also, the criteria used by Bradshaw and Gibbs' assessors are ambiguous and different conclusions might have emerged from other forms of assessment.)

It is probably the stigma which is attached to admission which explains why zero or near zero prices have led to only a moderate increase in expressed demand. Most elderly people view admission to a care home as something to be avoided if at all possible (RICA, 1988). There seems little doubt, however, that the impact on demand would be very much greater if 'vouchers' were made available in the same sort of way for care services delivered in people's own homes.

■ The 1990 NHS and Community Care Act

The beginning of the end for Income Support funding of residential and nursing home care for elderly people was signalled in 1986 with the publication of the Audit Commission report on community care (HMSO, 1986), which contained a scathing indictment of the failure of government, both central and local, to implement the policy of community care. Immediately afterwards the government invited Sir Roy Griffiths to conduct an inquiry, the report of which was published in 1988 (HMSO, 1988a). The central thrust of the Griffiths report was its proposal to make local authorities the lead agency for state financing of care services and to strengthen management accountability in pursuing the goal of community care. The principal financial recommendation was that the *care* element of Income Support funding of residential and nursing homes should be transferred by central government to local authorities, which would use the enlarged budget at their discretion to pay either for care in care homes or for home care services.

Most of Griffiths' recommendations were incorporated in the 1990 National Health Service and Community Care Act, the main community care provisions of which were implemented in April 1993, when local authorities became the principal budget-holders for state-funded long-term care. Reduced to its essentials, the new state financing structure replaces non-cash-limited, non-needs-tested social security funding for individuals entering care homes with cash-limited grants to be added to local authorities' existing grant allocation and local tax revenue and allocated according to need by local authorities both for residential and nursing home care and for care services for people living in their own homes.

For three financial years, 1993/94, 1994/95 and 1995/96, local authorities will receive a Special Transitional Grant from central government, the amounts of which are set out in *Table 2*, in addition to their ordinary personal social services allocations which are channelled through the Revenue Support Grant on the basis of Standard Spending Assessments (SSAs). The Special Transitional Grant, which will be 'ring-fenced' for spending on community care, will consist of what has become known as the 'social security transfer', representing the 'care' element of Income Support money that would have been claimed by new residents of residential and nursing homes if the old Income Support funding system had been retained. The 'non-care' or 'hotel' element of Income Support funding has not been transferred to local authorities because elderly residents of care homes still are able to claim the ordinary level of Income Support, together with the new Residential Allowance, from the Department of Social Security.

Table 2 Cumulative social security transfer to local authorities (£ million)

	1993/94	1994/95	1995/96
England local authorities	399.0[a]	1 050.0	1 568.0
England NHS[b]	5.0	6.0	6.0
Scotland	41.0	106.0	158.0
Wales local authorities	28.0	73.0	108.0
Wales NHS[b]	0.3	0.4	0.4
Great Britain total	**472.0**	**1 235.0**	**1 841.0**

Notes: [a] The Special Transitional Grant in England will include an additional £140 million for implementation costs to bring it to a total of £539 million.

[b] Represents amounts to be transferred to the NHS in respect of the NHS responsibility for hospice care.

Preserved rights of existing care home residents

Most residents of independent care homes on 31 March 1993 have a preserved right to continue to receive the old higher rate of Income Support, up to limits which will continue to be set annually by the Department of Social Security (DSS). The number of residents with preserved rights will decline as those individuals move out or die.

State benefits for new care home residents after April 1993

Since April 1993, the higher rate of Income Support has not been available for new entrants into care homes, though like anyone else they are entitled to ordinary Income Support payments, including any premiums, from the DSS if they pass the usual means test. Residents of independent care homes may also claim the new means-tested Residential Allowance as part of Income Support from the DSS. The Residential Allowance at April 1993 is £45 per week and slightly higher in London.

From April 1993 state-funded residents lose their entitlement to Attendance Allowance or the care component of Disability Living Allowance four weeks after admission. Privately paying residents, however, can continue to receive these benefits.

Assessment

With the exception of those people placed in nursing homes directly by health authorities, people wishing to enter a residential or nursing home at the public expense must approach their local social services authority for an assessment of their needs.

If assessment leads to a placement in a care home, the local authority will pay the full care home fee and recover a charge from the resident according to his or her means. If the individual is entitled to social security benefits, this will be counted as part of the resident's income in determining the charge to be paid, and this should ensure that benefit entitlements are actually claimed. There is provision for those residents or families who wish to pay the charge direct to the care home to be able to do so if the local authority and the care home agree. The local authority is, however, the contracting party with the care home, and even if the resident fails to pay his or her charge, the local authority will still be obliged to pay the full contracted fee.

People are free to choose to enter any residential or nursing home in the UK, subject to certain conditions. If the home costs more than the local authority would normally pay for someone with those assessed needs, the local authority will expect to collect the difference from the person or a third party.

▬ Concerns about the April 1993 reforms

The reforms undoubtedly provide a more rational framework for financing long-term care than existed prior to April 1993. There are, however, a number of concerns about the new system.

Though the right of state-funded individuals to enter a care home of their choice and have their fees topped up, provided they can afford to do so, has been secured by a statutory direction, there remains concern about the choice offered to state-funded users of services for people living in their own homes. Personal choice may be inhibited by the purchasing styles of local authorities or indeed any large organisation.

Approaches to empowering elderly consumers of state-funded care services are discussed in Chapter 7.

One of the primary objectives of the state funding changes introduced in April 1993 (apart from cash-limiting community care services) was to end perverse incentives to place people in residential or nursing homes rather than providing domiciliary services. To a large extent this objective has been achieved. It will usually be in the financial interest of a local authority to provide domiciliary services rather than place an elderly person in a residential or nursing home if the cost of the domiciliary services is less than the care home costs that the local authority has to meet. However, a perverse incentive still remains, as a consequence of means-testing. The greater the elderly person's means, the higher the charge the local authority may levy for residential or nursing home care. In some cases, the local authority will recover the whole of its costs in this way. Domiciliary services, on the other hand, are not subject to national means-testing rules. Though the government encourages local authorities to recover as much as they can in charges for domiciliary services, the fact is that local authority domiciliary charges recover only a small proportion of the cost of the service, and are likely to continue to do so in the future. In many cases under the new system, the net cost to the local authority of supporting a person in his or her own home may therefore be substantially greater than the net cost of buying the same amount of care in a care home. The objective of financial neutrality between the purchase of care in care homes and for people living in their own homes is not, therefore, entirely achieved by the new system. Whether this will have any practical impact on the care packages recommended for people whose assessment shows them to be on the margin of domiciliary care and care home admission remains to be seen.

The other perverse incentive (or absence of financial neutrality) within the new system is that residents placed in local authorities' own Part III accommodation will not be eligible for the new Residential Allowance. This provision was introduced deliberately by the government in order to deter local authorities from expanding their own in-house services with the transferred funding. The result is a strong incentive for local authorities to dispose of some or all of their Part III accommodation.

Adequacy of social security transfers

The main concern about the new state financing system is whether resources will be sufficient to maintain access to long-term care services at their present levels. The House of Commons Health Committee accepted that the Department of Health had ensured the transparency of its formula for distribution of the Transitional Grant, but argued that the assumptions underlying the formula were not clear (*Community Care: Funding from April 1993*, House of Commons Session 1992–93, 309–1, March 1993). It is now widely recognised amongst those involved in delivering care services that there are only limited opportunities for savings by substitution of domiciliary services and day care for residential and nursing home care at the margin. Resources will certainly have to be increased in order to cope with the pressures from demographic change.

At the time of writing, there are too many unknown factors to judge whether the social security transfer sums distributed by the government to local authorities will prove to be sufficient in the short term. In the medium and longer term, because spending will be progressively more cash-limited under the new regime, state funding for elderly care will almost certainly grow less rapidly than in the previous decade.

3 Who pays for long-term care in the UK?

The latest available estimates of state and personal spending on long-term care in the UK, annualised at April 1992, are set out in *Table 3*. They relate to the administrative arrangements in place prior to the April 1993 transfer of the care element of Income Support funding to local authorities. The broad pattern of state/personal financing has not, however, altered substantially. The shifts in state/personal spending patterns that the new state funding system will give rise to are discussed below. *Table 3* is constructed from a wide variety of sources. The broad principles on which estimates were made, and the derivation of some of the less readily accessible statistics on personal spending, are briefly summarised in the footnotes.

Total national spending on long-term care services, both in NHS and care home settings and for people living in their own homes, is estimated at £10.2 billion. These figures cover both elderly people (65 and over) and physically handicapped people under the age of 65. For elderly people only, estimated total national spending is £9.1 billion, 70 per cent of which is state-funded and the remaining 30 per cent personally funded, including user charges for state-supplied services.

National spending on long-term care services accounts for an estimated 1.65 per cent of GDP as at April 1992, for elderly and younger physically handicapped people combined. For elderly people only, the estimate is 1.47 per cent.

All these figures exclude the value of care provided by unpaid carers. *Table 3* also includes an estimate of the massive scale of such care, derived by applying local authority home help/home care worker pay rates to the hours of care provided by family and friends.

Table 3   Sources of finance for long-term care of elderly and physically disabled people (including psychogeriatric care but excluding all other psychiatric care), annualised UK estimates April 1992

CARE IN NHS AND CARE HOME SETTINGS	Aged <65 £ million	Aged 65+ £ million	All ages £ million	All ages %
NHS expenditure on NHS geriatric/ psychogeriatric beds	29	1 467	1 496	21
NHS expenditure on NHS beds for younger physically handicapped people (not in geriatric/psychogeriatric wards)	123	0	123	2
NHS expenditure on independent nursing homes	14	83	97	1
Total gross NHS expenditure on long-stay care in hospitals and nursing homes	166	1 550	1 716	24
less user charges	(0)	(0)	(0)	(0)
Net NHS expenditure on long-stay care in hospitals and nursing homes	166	1 550	1 716	24
Local authority expenditure on Part III homes	43	1 047	1 090	15
Local authority expenditure on independent residential and nursing homes	49	79	129	2
Gross local authority expenditure on residential and nursing homes	92	1 126	1 218	17
less user charges	(26)	(319)	(345)	(5)
Net local authority expenditure on residential and nursing homes	66	807	873	12
Income Support expenditure on independent care homes	134	2 009	2 143	30
Total net public expenditure on care in NHS and care home settings	366	4 366	4 732	66
User charges	26	319	345	5
Total personal expenditure on independent care homes	132	1 927	2 059	29
Total public and personal expenditure on care in NHS and care home settings	**524**	**6 612**	**7 136**	**100**

CARE FOR PEOPLE LIVING IN THEIR OWN HOMES	Aged <65 £ million	Aged 65+ £ million	All ages £ million	All ages %
NHS expenditure on care for people living in their own homes (community health)				
– district nursing	222	669	891	29
– day care	16	51	67	2
– chiropody	8	71	79	3
Total gross NHS expenditure on care for people living in their own homes	246	791	1 037	34
less user charges	(0)	(0)	(0)	(0)
Net NHS expenditure on care for people living in their own homes	246	791	1 037	34
Local authority expenditure on care for people living in their own homes				
– home care	114	701	815	16
– social work (estimate for elderly and physically handicapped clients)	55	238	293	9
– elderly day care (local authority and other provision)	0	130	130	4
– day care for younger physically handicapped	NA	0	NA	NA
– meals on wheels	0	90	90	3
– other elderly support services	0	85	85	3
– aids and adaptations	32	42	74	2
Total gross local authority expenditure on care for people living in their own homes	201	1 286	1 487	48
less user charges	(17)	(107)	(124)	(4)
Net local authority expenditure on care for people living in their own homes	184	1 179	1 363	44
Total net public expenditure on care for people living in their own homes	430	1 970	2 400	78
User charges	17	107	124	4
Other personal expenditure on care for people living in their own homes				
– aids and adaptations	63	83	146	5
– home care	79	343	422	14
Total public and personal expenditure on care for people living in their own homes	**589**	**2 503**	**3 092**	**100**

	Aged <65 £ million	Aged 65+ £ million	All ages £ million	All ages %
TOTAL LONG-TERM CARE EXPENDITURE				
– public sector spending	796	6 336	7 132	70
– user charges for public sector services	43	426	469	5
– other personal expenditure	274	2 353	2 627	26
ALL SOURCES OF FUNDING	1 113	9 115	10 228	100
CARE PROVIDED BY UNPAID CARERS[a]	[6 600]	[32 500]	[39 100]	[NA]
SOCIAL SECURITY PAYMENTS (1992–93)[b]				
– Attendance Allowance	0	1 202	1 202	NA
– Disability Living Allowance	1 676	336	2 012	NA
– Invalid Care Allowance	101[c]	200[c]	301	NA
– Independent Living Fund	NA	NA	97	NA

Notes: [a] Calculated following a method originally used by the Family Policy Studies Centre (1989), valuing each hour of care at £7 per hour (based on local authority pay rates).

[b] Relevant transfer payments are benefits specifically targeted at disabled individuals. To the extent that these benefits are spent on care services, they are included in 'personal expenditure' items above.

[c] Age of cared for person.

Source: Estimates from a number of public and private data sources, projected where necessary from England, England and Wales or Great Britain to UK level according to population ratios and projected where necessary to April 1992 by (a) applying a 'dependency index' derived from age-specific usage of long-term care in NHS and care home settings to take account of increasing utilisation owing to demographic change and (b) by applying the Department of Employment earnings index to adjust for service price changes. Personal spending on residential and nursing home care services is derived by subtracting state spending from estimated total spending (Laing and Buisson, 1993a). Personal spending on care services for people living in their own homes is estimated from data published by Martin and White (1988) in their OPCS study of the financial circumstances of disabled adults living in private households. Average spending on 'aids and adaptations' and on 'home services' among the OPCS sample was grossed up to UK level on the basis of population and projected forward from 1985 (when the OPCS fieldwork took place) to April 1992 using the dependency index and average earnings index methods summarised above.

The principal features of the UK system of long-term care financing are set out below, dealing in turn with expenditure on care in NHS and care home settings, expenditure on care services for people living in their own homes, and care provided by unpaid carers.

■ Who pays for care in NHS and care home settings?

Spending on long-term care for elderly people in NHS and care home settings is estimated at £6.6 billion in the UK in 1992, representing 73 per cent of the total spent on all long-term care services combined. State spending accounted for 66 per cent of the total for care in NHS and care home settings, the remaining 34 per cent coming from user charges (for local authority Part III homes), personal contributions from care home residents receiving Income Support, Income Support top-ups, and purely private care home fees.

With the exception of those people for whom the NHS accepts financial responsibility, all state-funded care for people outside their homes in the UK is means-tested. Elderly individuals entering such care must exhaust all their non-disregarded income and assets in excess of £8,000 before becoming eligible for state support from local authorities or from the Department of Social Security. The value of any owner-occupied property in which the resident formerly lived counts as an asset, unless it is still occupied by a partner, a relative who is aged 60 or over or incapacitated or, at the local authority's discretion, a carer (Department of Health, 1992). This is an exception to the usual rule that home equity is disregarded in determining eligibility for means-tested social security benefits, but it is in line with means-testing rules for long-term care outside people's own homes in most other countries (see Chapter 5). The rationale is that entry into a care home is generally permanent and thus the claimant has no need for his or her former home.

There are rules against divestment of assets with the aim of circumventing the means test, though the waiting period after divestment is much shorter than it is, for example, for people seeking to avoid Inheritance Tax. Under Section 21 of the Health and Social Services Adjudications (HASSASSA) Act 1983, a local authority may recover from a third party any assets which have been transferred at less than their value to that third party while the transferor is resident in a care home or within the previous six months. The divestment rules which apply for eligibility for Income Support are somewhat different and are not time-limited. Section 22 of the HASSASSA Act empowers local authorities to place a charge on property with a view to recovering any sums owed for residential or nursing home care when the property is sold, while Section 24 allows the local authority to charge a reasonable rate of interest on any outstanding sums.

The exception to these severe means-testing rules for state funding of long-term care outside people's own homes is NHS long-stay care, provided in NHS hospitals and in independent nursing homes under contract to a health authority. To the extent that NHS long-stay care is available, it is provided regardless of ability to pay and no charges are levied by the NHS. NHS patients receiving state contributory benefits have them reduced by 40 per cent after six weeks in hospital, and after a year they are further reduced to an amount sufficient for personal expenses, but patients do not have to spend other personal income such as occupational pensions or investment earnings and they do not have to spend down their assets to pay for long-stay NHS care. When viewed in the context of means-tested state funding of all other forms of long-term care outside people's own homes, this is something of an anomaly though, in view of the Prime Minister's pledge against privatisation of the NHS in the 1992 election campaign, there would be strong political objections to putting NHS long-stay care on the same footing as all other forms of care outside people's own homes. The NHS anomaly is, however, declining in importance as the scale of NHS long-stay provision shrinks, despite the acknowledged NHS duty to provide nursing care – in particular for those people who do not wish to be discharged into a fee-charging care home. It is estimated that NHS-funded residents, as a proportion of all people in long-term care in NHS and care home settings, have declined from 28 per cent in 1970 to 12 per cent in 1992. Surveys of health authorities' intentions indicate that the NHS share will decline further during the 1990s (Laing and Buisson, 1993a).

There is one very important detail of the local authority means-testing regime introduced in April 1993 which will lead to an immediate shift away from state funding and towards personal funding of long-term care outside people's own homes.

To understand the significance of the change, it is necessary to describe how the effects of the 1990–92 recession allowed large numbers of higher-rate Income Support claimants to slip through what at first sight appear to have been almost identical means-testing rules applied by social security offices – resulting in a significant move *towards* state funding and *away from* personal funding in the lead-up to April 1993.

It is well known that Income Support funding for care homes increased rapidly throughout the 1980s. What is less well known is that the period 1990–92 witnessed a remarkable ballooning of Income Support spending at the very time when the care element of the budget was about to be transferred to local authorities. This led to a major change in the financing profile of elderly and physically handicapped residents of independent care homes. The estimated proportion of residents in receipt of Income Support increased sharply from 48 per cent in February 1986 to 70 per cent in May 1992 (see *Table 4*).

It is believed, though no data are available to confirm this, that at least part of the explanation lies in the slump in the property market from the end of 1989. Elderly people who would normally have been able to sell their owner-occupied homes found themselves unable to sell and therefore eligible for Income Support on a temporary basis, thus increasing the overall number of claimants. Income Support regulations provided (and still provide) that where an individual has taken steps to realise the value of a property asset, but has not yet been able to achieve a sale, the value is disregarded when determining eligibility for Income Support for a period of six months. If the property is still unsold, the disregard may continue for another six months. Before April 1993, therefore, many people who were owner-occupiers on entry into an independent care home had a period of grace before Income Support was withdrawn. Though in many cases elderly people and their families were genuinely unable to sell property in a depressed market, it is possible that other owner-occupiers and their families became aware of the opportunity to receive Income Support funding and made full use of it in order to conserve assets.

The situation for such property owners changed completely from April 1993. Rather than disregarding the value of property which care home residents cannot realise, local authorities are empowered, as they have been for Part III and other supported residents in the past, to place a charge on residents' property and, after the property is sold, to recover, with interest, any sums owing from Day 1. As a result those owner-occupiers who, under the old Income Support system,

Table 4 Source of finance for residents in private and voluntary care homes, 1986–92

	Feb 1986	Nov 1988	May 1990	May 1991	Nov 1991	May 1992
Elderly and PH private payers						
– residents (000s)	76	94	111	95	86	83
– share of total (%)	46	41	40	32	28	26
Elderly and PH on Income Support (fees wholly or partly paid with Income Support)						
– residents (000s)	76	128	157	196	214	225
– share of total (%)	48	56	57	65	69	70
Elderly and PH NHS or local authority funded						
– residents (000s)	8	8	8	10	12	14
– share of total (%)	5	4	3	3	4	4
Total elderly and PH						
– residents (000s)	160	230	276	301	312	322
– share of total (%)	100	100	100	100	100	100
Psychiatric residents on Income Support (000s)	14	28	32	35	39	46
Elderly and PH on Income Support (000s)	76	128	157	196	214	225
Total on Income Support (000s)	90	155	189	231	253	271

Note: PH = physically handicapped.

Source: Laing and Buisson, 1993a.

could have conserved their assets by claiming the higher rate of Income Support for six months or more while their property was being sold will, under the post-April 1993 system, usually have no financial incentive to seek local authority support, since it will no longer be possible to conserve assets in this way. Since April 1993, property owners and their families seeking financial support from their local authority have had to consider whether it is in their financial interests to use the local authority as a 'banker'. Sometimes it is, when alternative liquid funds cannot be found. But in other cases families will prefer to make their own arrangements entirely outside the state funding system. The result will be a reversal of recent trends, a decrease in the proportion of long-term care outside people's own homes which is state-funded, and an increase in the number of elderly people paying privately.

As long as home equity is taken into account in means-testing rules, there will also be a longer-term trend away from state funding and towards personal funding of long-term care outside people's homes, as higher rates of home ownership filter through to members of the very old population most at risk of entering such care. According to *Table 3*, 34 per cent of all spending on long-term care in NHS and care home settings came from personal resources and 66 per cent from the state in 1992. It is possible that these ratios will be closer to 50:50 by the turn of the century.

■ Who pays for care for people living in their own homes?

Spending on long-term care for elderly people living in their own homes is estimated at £2.5 billion in the UK in 1992. State spending accounted for 79 per cent of this total, which is significantly higher than the share of long-term care in NHS and care home settings financed by the state – reflecting the less severe means-testing rules for care for people living in their own homes. The remaining 21 per cent comes from user charges for local authority domiciliary services and personal spending on private services.

Expenditure on care services for people living in their own homes provided by both health and local authorities has risen rapidly in real terms in the last decade. Official data from 1978/79 to 1989/90 are set out in *Table 5*. The geometric mean real increase for local authority services is 4.7 per cent per annum. This particular source does not give comparative figures for community health spending, but data published elsewhere show that spending on district nursing has also increased rapidly in real terms. The increase in real spending on long-term care services for people living in their own homes in the UK has almost certainly been greater than that necessary to keep pace with demographic change. There are no readily available statistics on age-specific usage of such services, but if it is in line with age-specific usage of care in NHS and care home settings, then a 2.5 per cent real annual increase would have been sufficient to keep pace with demographic change.

A similar spending comparison has not been attempted for long-term care in NHS and care home settings because of the unreliability of data on elderly people receiving long-stay NHS care and on the cost of that care.

Table 5 Expenditure in real terms^a on core community care services for elderly people, England 1978/79 and 1989/90

	1978/79 £ million	1989/90 £ million
LOCAL AUTHORITIES		
Home care (home helps/home care workers)	323	530
Meals on wheels	44	68
Aids and adaptations	29	46
Day care for elderly people	49	107
Local authority total^b	**440**	**731**
HEALTH AUTHORITIES		
General patient care (district nursing)	NA	535
Chiropody	NA	52
Other (non-psychiatric) day care	NA	44
Health authority total^b	**NA**	**631**

Note: ^a Real expenditure is derived by revaluing cash figures using the GDP deflator to average 1989/90 prices.
  ^b Expenditure on general social work and administration attributed to community care in *The Government's Expenditure Plans* has been omitted from this table.

Source: HMSO, 1992a.

In contrast with the major shifts in state financing of long-term care outside people's own homes, the framework for state financing of care services for elderly people living in their own homes has changed little in recent years. State-funded services for people living in their own homes are provided by both local authorities (home helps/home care workers, aids and adaptations, day care, meals on wheels and other support services) and health authorities, some of whose community health services are concentrated on elderly people with continuing care needs (in particular district nursing).

As with long-term care in NHS and care home settings, the funding principle for care services for people living in their own homes differs between health authorities (non-means-tested and free at the point of delivery) and local authorities (which may levy charges at their discretion). The position with local authority home helps/home care workers and other services for people living in their own homes is, however, complex. Local authorities are empowered to charge for their services under the 1983 HASSASSA Act, and the Conservative government's guidance (HMSO, 1993) is that local authorities should seek to recover the full economic cost of providing day and domiciliary services wherever this can be done without causing hardship to the user. Typically, local authorities recover only a small proportion of their gross expenditure from charges, but their charging policies vary widely.

There is little systematic information available, but there are two ways in which local authorities may target their domiciliary and day care resources selectively on those dependent elderly people without means of their own to pay for care. First, they may charge according to ability to pay, and this may involve taking account of benefits such as Attendance Allowance. Second, they may ration services by making them unavailable to any person with income above a certain level. It appears that many local authorities have recently sought to increase charges or to be more selective in their targeting.

'Informal selectivism'

By far the most important element of selectivism or means-testing in the distribution of state-funded care services for people living in their own homes is, however, non-financial. What may be termed 'informal selectivism' or 'informal means-testing' appears to be a guiding principle in the allocation of local authority care services. This refers to the well-attested finding that local authorities concentrate their domiciliary and day care resources on people who live alone and who do not have ready access to care provided by an unpaid carer. Those people who already have the support of a heavily involved carer, on the other hand, are typically left to cope by themselves, particularly if the carer is female and co-resident.

The results of the 1985 and 1990 General Household Surveys of carers graphically illustrate the skewed distribution of local authority services (see *Table 6*). In the case of home helps/home care workers, which account for the bulk of local authority spending on home care, 29 per cent of people whose carer lived elsewhere received regular home help in 1990. In contrast only 6 per cent of people with carers living in the same household did so. In the case of meals on wheels, the distribution was even more skewed with regular visits recorded by 9 per cent and 1 per cent respectively in 1990.

Table 6 Percentage of carers whose (main) dependant received regular visits, Great Britain, 1989 and 1990 (%)

	Carers whose (main) dependant lived			
	in the same household		in another private household	
	1985	1990	1985	1990
Doctor	13	8	26	19
Community or district nurse	14	13	16	16
Health visitor	5	3	6	5
Social worker	3	2	7	4
Home help/home care worker	7	6	30	29
Meals on wheels	1	1	10	9
Voluntary worker	1	2	5	4
Other	4	6	9	11
None of the above	69	73	46	49

Source: Green, 1988; Office of Population Censuses and Surveys (OPCS), 1992.

Twigg (1992), in her review of research and practice relating to carers, cites several studies from which similar conclusions have been drawn, whether based on small local surveys or on re-analysis of the 1985 General Household Survey results.

One of the most interesting points to emerge from the 1985 and 1990 General Household Survey results was that NHS community health services were delivered much more evenly than local authority domiciliary care services. The existence of carers living in the same household made little difference to the chance of receiving visits from either district nurses or health visitors. On this evidence, informal means-testing appears to be a particular inbuilt feature of local authority rationing, governed as it is by a selectivist ethos – in contrast with the universalist ethos of community health services, which appears to give rise to more equitable rationing.

Informal means-testing selects against certain classes of carer rather than against certain recipients of care, the criterion for selection being the availability of care provided by an unpaid carer rather than the availability of income or assets. In all other respects, however, the principle of 'informal selectivism' on which local authority domiciliary services are usually based very closely parallels the financial selectivism of local authority-funded residential and nursing home care, and raises precisely the same equity issues as the more familiar concept of financial selectivism.

▪ Care provided by unpaid carers

Table 3 gives the annualised value of care provided by unpaid carers at April 1992 as £39.1 billion for elderly people and younger physically handicapped people combined. For elderly people only, the figure is £32.5 billion. These calculations follow a method originally used by the Family Policy Studies Centre (1989), which in turn used data from Green's (1988) General Household Survey report on carers in Britain. Green's fieldwork took place in 1985, and the fieldwork for the subsequent OPCS follow-up took place in 1990. The number of hours of care provided by unpaid carers has been adjusted to 1992 by applying a 'dependency index' based on age-specific usage of long-term care in NHS and care home settings, to take account of demographic changes between 1990 and 1992. Each hour of care provided by unpaid carers has been valued at £7 per hour, based on local authority spending on home helps/home care workers per hour of service. The use of £7 per hour is appropriate for some purposes, but not for others. The importance of the calculation is not to make an all-purpose estimate of the 'value' of care provided by unpaid carers, but to demonstrate that it is very large indeed and that even a small withdrawal of family and friends from the care obligations they now accept would have very serious consequences for the amount of care that the state, or elderly individuals themselves, would have to pay for.

The burden of care is not spread evenly and can be very severe indeed for those individuals involved. This is best illustrated by data from the OPCS Retirement Survey (Bone et al, 1992) conducted in 1988 and early 1989 on behalf of the Department of Social Security. The survey, which covered the 55–69 age group only, used questions to identify carers which were almost identical to the General Household Survey of carers (Green, 1988). Seven per cent of those in the sample were caring for someone else in the same household while 13 per cent were caring for someone outside their own household. Co-resident carers devote the most time to caring and they also care for the longest durations. The median duration was seven years but 19 per cent had been caring for 20 or more years (*Figure 3*). These very long durations usually involve caring for people who became disabled while young, rather than frail elderly people. But the conclusion remains the same, that caring – whether for elderly people, physically handicapped people or mentally handicapped people – imposes a very heavy burden on a significant minority of people who provide care.

■ Social security payments

Apart from local and health authority spending on services, the other source of state funding for long-term care is social security payments to individuals, whether disabled people or their carers.

Attendance Allowance

Attendance Allowance, originally introduced in 1971, is a tax-free, non-means-tested, non-contributory benefit which is payable to people who are severely disabled, physically or mentally, and require help with personal care, supervision, or to have someone watching over them. As a non-means-tested benefit, its introduction was counter to the trend towards increasingly selective targeting of state

Figure 3 Number of years carers aged 55–69 spend caring

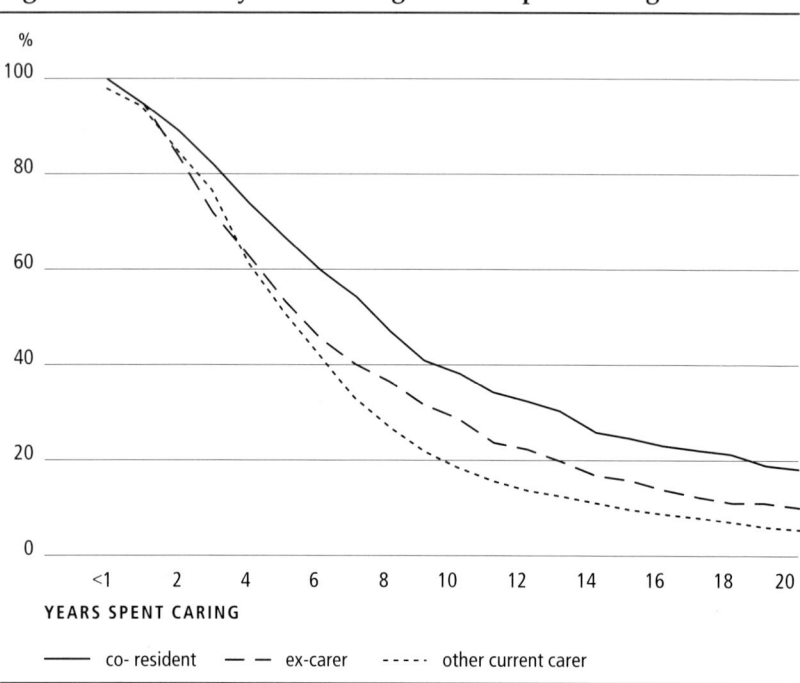

YEARS SPENT CARING

—— co-resident   — — ex-carer   - - - - - other current carer

Source: Bone et al, 1992.

funding on people without adequate resources of their own, which has been a feature of the postwar development of long-term care services for dependent elderly people. Attendance Allowance is paid at a higher or lower rate, depending on the amount of care deemed to be required. It is available both to people living in private households and to people living in care homes, though from April 1993 it is discontinued after four weeks for all local authority-funded care home residents and those who claim Income Support. Self-paying care home residents can still receive Attendance Allowance. In April 1992, Attendance Allowance was replaced by Disability Living Allowance for those people disabled before the age of 65. For the remaining people entitled to Attendance Allowance, aged 65 and over, an estimated £1,208 million in benefits was paid in the UK in the financial year 1992/93 (see *Table 3*). No official analysis of the type of beneficiary is available, but on the assumption that 250,000 residents of care homes were receiving Attendance Allowance at the higher rate, long-term care outside people's own homes would have absorbed an annualised equivalent of £540 million at April 1992. This figure will drop substantially from April 1993.

From the assumptions set out above, it follows that an estimated £660 million of Attendance Allowance would have been available in 1992/93 to help disabled elderly people living in private households.

Disability Living Allowance

Disability Living Allowance was introduced in April 1992. Like Attendance Allowance, it is tax-free, non-means-tested and non-contributory. It replaced Attendance Allowance for those who become disabled before the age of 65, and it replaced Mobility Allowance entirely. Entitlement is split into a care component (three rates) and a mobility component (two rates). People who become disabled before the age of 65 are entitled to continue receiving Disability Living Allowance after the age of 65, as was the case with Mobility Allowance previously.

Given that 28 per cent of Mobility Allowance benefits were being paid to people aged 65 or over prior to its replacement by Disability Living Allowance, it can be estimated that about £340 million in Disability Living Allowance benefits was paid to people aged 65 and over in 1992/93 (see *Table 3*).

On the assumption that most, if not almost all, Disability Living Allowance is paid to individuals living in private households, it can be estimated that a total of about £1,000 million from Attendance Allowance and Disability Living Allowance combined was available for spending by disabled elderly people in private households in 1992/93. Only about half of this, however, appears to be spent on care services. It is estimated in *Table 3* that personal expenditure on care services and aids and adaptations by elderly disabled people living in private households amounted to some £533 million, about four-fifths on private services and the remaining one-fifth on local authority charges.

Invalid Care Allowance

Benefits for carers also help to finance care services. Invalid Care Allowance is the only benefit specifically targeted at individuals who spend substantial amounts of time looking after a disabled person. Invalid Care Allowance is a non-contributory benefit, but it is effectively means-tested because it is available only for men and women under pension age who are not earning more than a specified amount and who look after a severely disabled person for at least 35 hours a week. The severely disabled person must be receiving either Attendance Allowance or the higher or middle rate of the care component of Disability Living Allowance or Constant Attendance Allowance paid with an industrial, war or service pension. The recipient is also credited with Class 1 National Insurance contributions, which is essential to protect the carer's entitlement to a retirement pension and other contributory National Insurance benefits. Because of the restrictive rules on entitlement, only a small proportion of carers receive Invalid Care Allowance. In 1991, 159,000 carers in Britain were receiving this benefit, compared with an estimated total number of carers of some 6.8 million. McLaughlin (1992) estimates that about one in ten carers providing around 35 hours of care per week receives Invalid Care Allowance.

Independent Living Fund

A novel recent experiment in state funding of care has been the Independent Living Fund. This was set up by the government in 1988 to help people with disabilities to live in the community. It provided money on a discretionary basis – frequently substantial sums – tailored case by case but spent by the individuals themselves. The budget was, however, comparatively small, at £97 million in 1992/93, and most of the spending was on younger physically disabled people rather than elderly people. In the summer of 1990 eligibility was restricted to people under 75, though this restriction was lifted in March 1991. As part of the community care reforms, the Independent Living Fund closed to new applications in November 1992 and was wound up in March 1993, with a successor trust taking over payments to existing beneficiaries from April 1993. At the same time a new fund was set up to work alongside local authorities in helping people aged 16–64 with the most severe disabilities to live independently in the community. Elderly people are specifically excluded from benefiting. With the demise of the Independent Living Fund, the most important state-sponsored experiment to date in financial empowerment of elderly disabled people, providing them with substantial sums to spend at their own discretion, has come to an end.

Income Support

Income Support is a means-tested benefit which is calculated as the difference between what the government says an individual needs each week and the individual's weekly income, excluding certain disregarded parts of income. Capital assets of over £8,000, excluding certain disregarded items, make an individual ineligible for Income Support. Up until April 1993 anyone could, subject to their means, claim a special higher rate of Income Support if they entered an independent residential or nursing home; the government set national weekly limits according to the type of care provided. Income Support (previously Supplementary Benefit) used also to be available to pay for private domestic help for people living in ordinary households, but this was abolished under the 1986 Social Security Act.

The higher rate of Income Support is now available only to people with preserved rights, who were already living in independent care homes on 31 March 1993. The ordinary rate of Income Support, however, together with the various premiums, is still an important source of funding for care services for people living in their own homes.

▪ Unresolved issues in state financing

A major unresolved issue is how much long-stay nursing care the NHS should pay for. It has been noted that the volume of NHS provision has been declining and is projected to decrease further in the future. It has also been noted that this implies a shift from non-means-tested NHS provision to means-tested alternatives, which some commentators have viewed as a denial of the proper responsibilities of the NHS. The fourth report of the Social Security Committee (HMSO, 1991) identifies the nub of the issue, reiterating the unequivocal Department of Health acceptance that:

> Health authorities have a responsibility under the National Health Service Act 1977 to provide nursing care for those who cannot or do not wish to pay for it. Department of Health guidance is clear that people should not be discharged into private nursing homes if they have no wish to pay.

In practice, however, according to the Committee's report, some hospitals fail to follow the guidance and put pressure on relatives and patients to accept discharge into a residential or nursing home without fully explaining that they then become liable for the costs of care. Hospitals may also inappropriately discharge elderly patients into their own homes, leaving relatives to arrange admission into a residential or nursing home.

The question at the heart of this controversy is one of fairness. Elderly patients and their relatives may feel they have been unfairly denied access to comprehensive health care which they thought they had paid for through their taxes. The counter-argument, however, is that it is inequitable that those elderly people needing long-term care outside their own homes who happen to find themselves in a long-stay NHS bed pay nothing, while the great majority who are in other forms of long-term care outside their own homes are liable to pay until their resources are exhausted and they can claim state support from local authorities and the Department of Social Security.

Apart from the question of fairness, any further withdrawal of the NHS from funding long-stay care raises the spectre of conflict between health and local authorities because, since April 1993, care responsibilities shed by the NHS have to be picked up by local authorities.

A second, broader issue concerns the appropriateness of selectively targeting state resources on people without resources of their own, which was established as the main state financing principle for long-term care in 1948 and has been reinforced in most funding changes since. Chapter 7 considers the case for an alternative, non-means-tested social insurance model of state financing and Chapter 5 identifies other OECD countries which have wholly or partly adopted such a model.

A third issue relates to the merits of a budget-capped system of state financing which depends on priority-setting and rationing by budget-holders (that is, local authorities), with no clearly stated entitlements to care services based on objective measures of dependency. Under tight financial constraints, budget-holders tend to target resources on those people with the highest dependency levels, leaving those with a lower level of dependency with nothing. It may be asked whether this is a fair way to distribute resources.

A fourth and related issue concerns choice and the empowerment of consumers of state-funded services, and is discussed in more detail in Chapter 7. The government's decision to issue statutory guidance to local authorities requiring them to offer people a choice of care home did much to allay fears of possible abuse of bureaucratic powers in relation to care homes. There remains concern, however, that no similar steps have been taken to promote genuine responsiveness to user preferences for packages of care for people living in their own homes. The government's approach to financing care services for people living in their own homes is in this sense at odds with its own philosophy. One of the main strands of current government policy is the creation of new administrative arrangements which place purchasing power as close as possible to the consumers of services, whether through practice funds for general practitioners, provisions for schools to opt out of local authority control, or the right of council tenants to buy their own homes or choose an alternative manager for their council estate. As far as long-term care for people living in their own homes is concerned, the issue of how to promote user choice has not yet been seriously addressed at central government level.

Finally, there is the issue of how state financing should relate to private financing of long-term care. Is there scope for financial products which complement state benefits? Should taxation and Inland Revenue regulations be amended to encourage the development of appropriate private funding mechanisms? These questions are also considered in Chapter 7.

4 Personal payment for long-term care

Table 7 shows the overall balance of public and private financing of long-term care, taking all sources of payment into account. It is estimated that, in April 1992, 34 per cent of the cost of all care in NHS and care home settings came from personal spending. For care for people living in their own homes, personal funding accounts for only 21 per cent of all spending. Data are insufficiently reliable to track any shift between state and personal funding in recent years.

Table 7 Segmentation of public and private expenditure on long-term care of elderly people, UK, April 1992 (%)

	Care in NHS and care home settings	Care for people living in their own homes	Total
Public finance/public supply[a]	33	78	45
Public finance/independent supply[b]	33	1	24
Personal finance/public supply[c]	5	4	5
Personal finance/independent supply[d]	29	17	26
	100	100	100

Note: [a] Local authority net revenue expenditure on care homes and domiciliary care and NHS expenditure on long-stay geriatric, psychogeriatric and younger physically disabled in-patients and day care services.

[b] DSS Income Support, NHS contracts and local authority contracts with independent providers of care homes and domiciliary care.

[c] Local authority charges.

[d] Personally paid fees to independent care homes and home care providers.

Source: Derived from *Table 3*.

■ Current sources of personal finance for residential and nursing home care

According to *Table 3*, in 1992 an estimated £2.2 billion of personal income and wealth was spent on long-term care for people aged over 65 in residential and nursing homes. Probably about £1.3 billion of this was spent on private care entirely outside the state funding system, while the remaining £0.9 billion represents personal contributions to state-funded services.

Because entry into a care home is rarely a planned event, money has to be found at fairly short notice. If the elderly person is not eligible for Income Support, savings may be used and relatives may contribute. If the elderly person was living alone in his or her own owner-occupied home, then release of the capital tied up in the (no longer occupied) home will typically be the first option considered to finance the cost of care over the long term. Elderly people rarely arrange admission to a care home themselves. Relatives are usually the prime movers and are usually intimately involved in financial decisions. Sensitive questions on inheritance and how to make use of house equity and other savings may then arise.

It is believed that house equity is the largest source of private funding for nursing and residential home care and, though no direct statistical confirmation is available, some indirect supporting evidence is cited in a recent study of inheritance sponsored by PPP Lifetime. The author (Hamnett, 1992) points out that:

> Given the growth in home ownership rates over the last 60 years, it would be expected that the number of estates passing at death containing house property would have shown a steady growth over the last 20 years, even though most of the post war home buyers will still be alive. But in reality the number has remained stable at about 145,000 since the late 1960s. This suggests that countervailing factors may be at work.

The principal countervailing factor identified by Hamnett is the sale of housing assets in order to pay for care.

■ Current sources of personal finance for care for people living in their own homes

According to *Table 3*, in 1992 something over £500 million of personal income was spent on long-term care for people aged 65 and over living in their own homes. About £400 million of this was spent on private care entirely outside the state funding system, while the remaining £100 million represents charges for local authority services. Oldman (1991), who has reviewed the market for private care services, found little hard information about how this money is spent. Probably, most of the £400 million is spent on services provided on a cash basis.

Results from the OPCS Disability Survey (Martin and White, 1988), on which the spending estimates in *Table 3* are based, indicate that the private market consists of large numbers of elderly people spending small amounts on care services. The most severely disabled respondents (OPCS categories 9 and 10) spent the most, but still a surprisingly low average of £2.60 per week in 1985 when the survey was carried out.

Professor Roy Parker has argued, on the basis of Family Expenditure Survey data, that there is a considerable amount of small-scale, paid *domestic* help for elderly people, provided by women working part-time on a cash basis. He estimates that about 1 million retired households in the UK purchased private domestic help during the two weeks of the 1986 Family Expenditure Survey (Sinclair et al, 1990).

The amount of care that individuals purchase from commercial agencies is believed to be relatively small, though money originating from the Independent Living Fund has led to increased use of commercial agencies in recent years. Hard figures do not exist. The private home care sector now has a representative organisation, the UK Home Care Association (UKHCA), set up in 1990. It has approaching 200 members – mainly small businesses. A survey of members of the UKHCA found that the pattern of service they provide contrasts strongly with that provided in the public sector. Whereas social service departments provide an average of three hours per week to their clients, members of the UKCHA were typically providing 25–40 hours

---

58

per week to theirs or even more (Johnstone, 1991). Home care agencies thus seem to be specialising in providing highly intensive care services. One reason may be that customers who need only a few hours care per week, and cannot get it through social services, find it easier and cheaper to make use of care providers working on a cash basis. The attractions of care agencies are stronger when there is a substantial requirement for regular care.

The absence of an organised, commercial home care sector in Britain on any significant scale contrasts with the large-scale (though still fragmented) commercial residential and nursing home sector. The main reason, as noted by both Oldman and Parker, is that home care has a high labour component and commercial organisations' overheads, in particular invoicing and payment collection, tend to make their prices uncompetitive compared with prices charged by individuals offering services on a cash basis with no VAT charged, few if any overheads, and usually no payment of National Insurance or income tax. The other reason is that the low-price, often subsidised home care service offered by local authorities has, despite its limitations, undercut commercial operators, and restricted their potential market to pure private payers or to those seeking care services to top up what they receive from local authorities.

Most commercial organisations currently believe that any significant development of a commercial home care sector will depend on third-party funding. The main potential source of such third-party funding at present is local authorities. The government's guidance that 85 per cent of the funding transferred from Income Support to local authority budgets for the year 1993/4 must be spent on the independent sector raises the prospect of a sharp stimulus to the commercial home care sector. The rule provides an additional stimulus for local authorities to contract out rather than develop their own in-house home care services.

In the longer term, the new long-term care financial products which are now emerging may also become a significant source of private third-party funding for long-term care services for people living in their own homes.

■ Future affordability of private long-term care funding products

If the private sector is to have a growing role in the financing of long-term care, as many commentators believe is inevitable, it is important to know to what extent the elderly population is able to pay, and how this is likely to change.

The following sections deal with trends in income and wealth. They focus specifically on the resources of the elderly generation itself because decisions to set money aside for long- term care will probably continue to be taken largely by people who are already retired or on the point of retirement, whether the present patchwork of private financing remains the norm or whether the new market for private financial products starts to take off.

The experience from the United States, which has the most highly developed market for long-term care funding products, is that long-term care insurance is typically bought by people who have already retired. It is rare for individuals to start prefunded long-term care schemes when they are young to middle-aged, and although employer-sponsored schemes are becoming more commonplace in the United States, they still account for a small proportion of long-term care insurance business.

Annuity, pseudo-annuity and equity release products for long-term care (see below) will also be purchased almost exclusively by elderly people in immediate need of care services. Even if pension products turn out to be the major source of private sector funding for long-term care, the crucial decision on how to apply the proceeds of the pension fund will not be taken during the individual's working lifetime but at the time of retirement in the light of competing claims on the available money at that time.

For these reasons the following discussion focuses on the ability to pay of elderly people themselves.

In the 1960s and 1970s, social scientists popularised a view of elderly people as an impoverished generation. In the 1980s, marketeers began to wake up to the potential scale of their purchasing power and developed a concept of the new, affluent elderly generation. The reality, in the 1990s, lies somewhere in between.

The economic situation of the current generations of elderly people can best be understood in terms of the times they lived through when younger, the provision made for the future through their employment, and the opportunities they have had for capital accumulation.

According to an analysis by Bosanquet et al (1990) there are three typical groups of older consumer in the UK:

- well-off older people, who are at a wealth and income peak at or near retirement – they account for about 20 per cent of households;

- retired middle-income households, which are often property-rich but income-poor – they account for about 40 per cent of households;

- elderly people (many living alone) who are mainly dependent on state benefits. This group is most at risk of poverty. They account for the remaining 40 per cent of households.

The outlook for the 1990s is that numbers of middle-income households will grow more rapidly than numbers of well-off households. Households of the first type, the well-off older people or 'WOOPIES', will only become prominent in the first two decades of the next century when the retirement of the baby boom generation will transform the economic situation of elderly people and create markets on a new scale to serve the ageing youth markets of the 1960s.

Some European countries are already a decade ahead of Britain as regards the economic status of their elderly population. An OECD study has found that the disposable income of households in the 65–74 age group across eight countries was 93 per cent of the average for all households, compared with 76 per cent for the UK (OECD, 1988b).

The two most important variable factors in determining the economic situation of succeeding generations of British elderly people, and their ability to pay personally for long-term care provision, are home ownership (as the principal form of personal wealth) and occupational and personal pensions (as the main contributor, alongside income from investment, to enhancing the incomes of elderly people in the future).

Home ownership in the elderly generation

The current elderly generation has participated to a substantial extent, but not yet fully, in the postwar growth in owner occupation. House ownership is the single most important form of wealth for about half the population of Britain. Capital from house sales is one of the most important sources of private funding for nursing and residential home care. This is possible because people entering a care home are predominantly those who have lost their spouse or have never had one. In the absence of any other co-resident family member or carer with ownership rights, the previous home of the person entering a care home is usually available for sale to finance future care. Though the depression in the housing market from 1990 to 1993 has made it difficult for prospective residents to realise their asset at an acceptable price, economic recovery will re-establish the primacy of property sale as a mechanism for private funding of nursing and residential home care. The long-term trend, unaffected by the recession, is for more elderly people to become owner-occupiers as high rates of home ownership among younger age groups feed through into the age band at risk of needing long-term care (see *Table 8*). In 1990, 54 per cent of heads of household in the 70–79 age bracket owned their own homes. They will be replaced in 20 years' time by those currently in the 45–59 age group, where the owner occupation rate was 77 per cent in 1990. Moreover, the great majority of older owner-occupiers have repaid their mortgages and own their property outright, making the capital fully available, in principle, to fund long-term care.

Owner occupation has filtered through to the least extent among very old single people living alone, who form the main clientele for long-term care services. According to the General Household Survey, 46 per cent of people aged 60 and over and living alone in 1990 owned their own homes (see *Table 8*). Analysis of how this percentage varies with age is hampered by small numbers at this level of subdivision, but unpublished data combining results from two previous years suggest that rates of owner occupation decline with age among single-person households, as among all types of household, to reach a floor of a little over 40 per cent for people aged 80 or over in 1990. In 20 years' time the corresponding figure may exceed 60 per cent (Barry, 1992).

Table 8 Owner occupation by age of head of household, Great Britain, 1990 (%)

AGE	Owned outright	Owned with mortgage	Total
<25	1	32	33
25–29	1	59	60
30–44	5	68	73
45–59	24	53	77
60–64	46	20	66
65–69	53	8	61
70–79	50	4	54
80+	51	2	53
single person aged 60+	42	4	46

Source: Smyth and Browne, 1992, *Tables 3.29(b)* and *3.34(b)*.

An indication of a potentially massive future increase in the use of house property to fund long-term care is provided by a forecasting model constructed to examine the impact of the growth of home ownership and changes in demographic structure on housing inheritance (Hamnett, 1992). The author calculates that, other things being equal, the projected number of properties inherited in Britain could grow from an average of 168,000 a year in the period 1986–91 to an average of 343,000 a year in the period 2026–31 (see *Table 9*). The author goes on to argue, however, that the scenario of mass housing inheritance which has been projected by many commentators is unlikely to become a reality, to the extent that house property will be sold to pay for long-term care or mortgaged to provide for income in old age. It is possible that property-owning families may increasingly seek to protect inheritances by early transfer of ownership, but there are drawbacks to such transfer and if it became widespread the government might bring in regulations to avoid it.

How much is this housing equity worth and how much long-term care could it finance? Building societies provide the most up-to-date private data source. Looking at data from Nationwide Anglia Building Society on realised house prices in different regions of the country, it is possible to conclude that substantial numbers of elderly people in the South-East and in affluent areas elsewhere in Britain occupy houses with a market value in excess of £100,000. Sums of this magnitude should usually be more than adequate to fund the cost of good-quality residential or nursing home care for life. Smaller sums would be sufficient to fund home care services, where individuals typically require less intensive services. Uptake of equity release mechanisms to pay for long-term care is still limited, but the Nationwide data suggest that the potential exists for more extensive personal financing of long-term care through such mechanisms, provided safe and efficient financial products become available to translate these resources into effective demand.

Table 9 Projected number of properties passing at death excluding spouse-to-spouse transfers, Britain, 1986–2031

YEAR	Number of properties (000s per annum)
1986–1991	168
1991–1996	188
1996–2001	207
2001–2006	227
2006–2011	246
2011–2016	269
2016–2021	291
2021–2026	318
2026–2031	343

Source: Hamnett, 1992.

Income of elderly households

The distribution of income among retired households, presented in *Table 10*, appears to indicate that few people can afford to pay for substantial amounts of care out of ordinary income. And few could potentially afford to make comprehensive provision out of ordinary income against the risk of needing long-term care in the future, for example by paying long-term care insurance premiums or by giving up some pension income at the start of retirement in return for augmented pension income in the event of needing care. As an illustration, the lowest price being quoted in 1991 for long-term care insurance with reasonably comprehensive benefits for residential or nursing home care was about £60 per week for a married couple at age 65, rising steeply with age. The second column of *Table 10* shows that only about the best-off one-fifth of one-man/one-woman retired households would have been able to cover premiums at this level without the cost of this single item exceeding 20 per cent of their normal gross income. This illustration confirms what most commentators believe: that affordability is, and will continue to be, a major constraint on the purchase of long-term care insurance in Britain.

Similar conclusions have been drawn in other countries. Weiner (1992a), using the Brookings-ICF Long-Term Care Financing Model, estimates on the basis of optimistic assumptions about willingness to pay that reasonably comprehensive long-term care insurance may be affordable by 20–32 per cent of elderly people in the United States. Most other studies in the USA have broadly confirmed these conclusions.

Table 10 Gross weekly income distribution of retired households, UK, 1991 (%)

£ PER WEEK	Retired single-person households	One-man, one-woman retired households
<60	23	0
60–79	18	1
80–99	15	8
100–124	14	14
125–149	7	14
150–174	5	12
175–224	6	16
225–274	4	10
275–324	3	8
325–374	2	5
375–424	1	3
425+	1	9
All incomes	100	100

Source: HMSO, 1992a.

What are the prospects for elderly people being better able to afford long-term care or long-term care insurance out of income in the future? The income of those close to and past retirement will depend in the future mainly upon the level and coverage of state and occupational pensions.

Unless there is a change of government and/or policy in Britain, the basic state pension will not be a source of increased income for elderly people generally during the 1990s. Britain, like a number of other OECD countries, has sought ways of limiting the cost of pensions to the state. One of the means used by Britain has been price indexation rather than earnings indexation. As long as this policy remains in place it will act as a brake on improvement of the financial situation of those elderly households mainly dependent on state benefits.

Much of the recent improvement in the incomes of elderly households has been due to occupational pensions. The proportion of people entitled to occupational pensions has increased significantly over the past 20 years, as has the average amount of occupational pension received (see *Table 11*). Just over half of newly retiring people now have occupational pensions. However, many of those covered still receive fairly small sums of money and many recipients lose a substantial proportion of the total value of the pension through an 'occupational pensions trap', whereby receipt of an occupational pension removes entitlement to state means-tested benefits.

Since membership of occupational pension schemes peaked at the end of the 1960s, the proportion of people receiving some pension will not continue to grow as it has done in the past 20 years. Whatever further enhancement there is of elderly people's incomes from this source will therefore come mainly from changes in the level of pension entitlement:

- Existing pensioners will be affected by policies on indexation of pensions: the outlook here is that existing occupational pensions will at best maintain their real value. If conditions worsen in stock markets they may not even do this.

- New pensioners will be affected by early retirement and by

Table 11 Proportion of retired people receiving occupational
pensions and average pension received, by year of birth,
sex and marital status

YEAR OF BIRTH	Men %	£ per week	Married women %	£ per week	Single/widowed women %	£ per week
1900–04	54	40	4	0	26	0
1905–09	56	45	5	34	30	30
1910–14	61	44	7	29	33	35
1915–19	67	57	11	29	40	35
1920–24	70	65	17	29	46	40
1925–29	0	0	22	31	49	47

Source: Johnson, 1992.

consequent loss of pension benefits following the employment
shake-out in the 1970s and 1980s.

- Single/widowed women will continue to benefit less than other
groups from occupational pensions. There is an improvement in
the pipeline for younger widows, who are increasingly likely to be
covered by their husbands' entitlements, but older widows will
continue to fare relatively badly.

The next significant boost to incomes from occupational pensions
will be from 1998 onwards, when people will be retiring with a full
SERPS entitlement after 20 years of contributions. However, the boost
will be less than envisaged when SERPS was originally introduced because of the significant downgrading of SERPS benefits under the 1986
Social Security Act, which reduced the proportion of average earnings
replaced from 25 per cent to 20 per cent, changed the 'best 20 years'
for calculating pension entitlement to the lifetime average (except in
certain circumstances for carers of children and adult dependants),
and reduced the portion of the pension inherited by a widow or wid-
ower from 100 per cent to 50 per cent.

On balance, therefore, the prospect for the remainder of the 1990s
seems to be limited improvements in the incomes of elderly people.
Robins and Wittenberg (1992), writing from the perspective of the
Economics and Operational Research Division of the Department of
Health, come to a similar conclusion. They note that 'It seems unlikely

that . . . rising real net incomes will result in elderly people contributing much more to the costs of their health care over the next 10 to 15 years'.

In the second and third decades of the twenty-first century, another boost will come when people with personal pensions bought in the 1980s start to retire. The introduction of personal pensions was the main new event on the pensions scene in the 1980s, with 3.5 million policies written in the UK. But virtually no personal pensions were sold to men over 50 or women over 45. This new form of saving will therefore have no impact on the economic position of people retiring in the 1990s.

In summary, therefore, the next 20 years will be a period of limited improvement in older people's ability to pay for long-term care out of income, or to afford financial products assuring long-term care. The major boost to older people's purchasing power is likely to come in the second decade of the next century, when the economically privileged baby boom generation retires.

During the same period, in contrast, elderly people's capacity to pay for residential or nursing home care through liquidation of home equity should increase significantly. As a result, the period may witness a shift away from the current 66:34 ratio of state funding to personal funding of long-term care outside people's own homes to something closer to 50:50.

These conclusions rest on fairly rudimentary analysis, taking account of the major economic and demographic trends likely to affect ability to pay. No full-scale simulation of personal ability to pay in the future has been undertaken in Britain. In the United States, however, Rivlin and Weiner (1988) have reported the results of the Brookings-ICF Long-Term Care Financing Model, which produces detailed projections of the number of disabled elderly people, their income, resources and likely use of long-term care. Many of the conclusions from this model are similar to those noted above for Britain, including the key conclusion that private sector products for financing long-term care are unlikely to be affordable by the large majority of elderly people.

■ Financial products for long-term care

This section contains a brief description of the new financial products for long-term care which have been launched on the market in the last two years. The case, if any, for changes in the tax environment and means-testing regime in order to stimulate the development of a choice of more effective and tax-efficient financial products is considered in Chapter 7.

Towards the end of the 1980s, the financial services sector started to look seriously at the challenge of developing products for financing long-term care. The reasons for this new interest were:

- ageing of the population;

- the view that the elderly population is becoming better off and more willing and able to pay for financial products for long-term care;

- the perception that the state will never provide anything more than a means-tested safety net for elderly care services with the middle and higher income groups left to look after themselves.

It was not until 1991 that the first financial products clearly packaged and designed for funding long-term care services were introduced on to the British market. There are five types of financial product, each potentially appealing to a different clientele. These can in turn be classified into two broad groups. The first group is made up of prefunded schemes such as long-term care insurance and pension-linked products, where the individual starts to pay while still fit and does not know whether he or she will need to claim. The second group consists of immediate care products such as annuities or equity release products, where the individual needs to finance care services immediately and typically pays a single premium.

The issue of whether long-term care is 'insurable' relates to the first, prefunded group of products. The main concerns are:

- Moral hazard: to the extent that the benefits trigger is under the control of the insured person, insurers may suffer from moral hazard – that is, increased use induced by insurance coverage.

- Adverse selection: if people can predict whether they will use long-term care services, those most in need of services may buy insurance disproportionately. This will drive use beyond expected levels and cause insurers to raise premiums. This in turn will cause low-risk people to drop their insurance, pushing average use and premiums still higher. To protect against adverse selection, insurers may screen for health problems and either exclude cover for pre-existing conditions or load premiums.

- The predictability of costs for the insured population as a whole: in this regard, long-term care insurance is a very risky product for insurers. Not only is there no British claims experience but unforeseen events in the 10, 20 or 30 years between the initial purchase of cover and eventual claims may cause claims experience to diverge dramatically from initial projections.

Personal pension products

The first UK long-term care funding product, 'Oasis Plus', launched by Cannon Lincoln in February 1991, took the form of an option on a standard personal pension plan whereby 10 per cent of the pension annuity income after retirement is forgone in return for a substantial increase in the pension annuity income if (a) the person is unable to carry out any four out of six Activities of Daily Living (ADLs) or (b) if he or she reaches the age of 85 regardless of state of health. The Inland Revenue, however, subsequently withdrew approval for these products, on the grounds that as age- or dependency-related enhancements are not allowed for occupational pensions they should not be allowed for personal pensions either.

In common with Cannon Lincoln, all other providers of long-term care funding products in Britain have chosen to use ADLs as a trigger for receipt of benefits. The advantages and disadvantages of ADLs are discussed at the end of this section.

Stand-alone long-term care insurance

Commercial Union launched the first such product in June 1991. Its 'Well-being' plan is aimed at individuals aged between 40 and 75.

Well-being offers benefits of up to £25,000 per annum, triggered by failing ADL conditions. There is a choice between Premier Cover for moderate and severe disability and Reserve Cover for severe disability only. Premier cover pays out 50 per cent of benefits on two ADLs (moderate disability – the person is likely to need home care) and 100 per cent on four ADLs (severe disability – the person is likely to need residential or nursing home care) or cognitive failure. Reserve cover pays out on four ADLs or cognitive failure only. Benefits are paid direct to the care provider in order to avoid income tax in the hands of the policyholder. Level monthly premiums or single premiums vary by age, sex and level of cover chosen and are subject to review. The policy lapses without value if premiums cease to be paid and no benefit is payable on death.

MGI Prime Health, a medical expenses insurer, launched its long-term care product in October 1991. This product is geared towards home care rather than residential or nursing home care and is unique in offering an option for home care only. It replaces the usual six ADLs with its own scale of 19 qualifying disabilities, allowing more finely graduated benefits. The home care benefits are defined in terms of hours of care instead of pounds per week. As with Commercial Union, benefits are paid direct to care providers in order to avoid income tax in the hands of the policyholder.

PPP Lifetime, a subsidiary of the medical insurance provident association PPP, has launched plans which, like others, use ADL triggers and make payments to care providers. A specific benefit to buy equipment or undertake house modifications is incorporated. PPP Lifetime also markets a 'dread disease' policy, aimed at younger people, which may be switched to a long-term care insurance plan at a later date.

Aetna launched its long-term care insurance policy in October 1991. Benefits are triggered by failure on two out of five ADLs and the chosen benefit scale is doubled if the claimant is admitted to a residential or nursing home on a doctor's recommendation. Aetna gives claimants the option of receiving the income themselves or paying the residential or nursing home or care provider direct. Aetna appears to have decided not to pursue the course of *contracting* direct with the care provider which other insurers maintain is the condition for avoiding taxation. The plan brochure states that the income payments are taxable under the current rules, whether received by the individual or paid direct to a care home.

Hambro Guardian has also launched a stand-alone long-term care insurance product but, unlike the other products, it is aimed at employers. The plan is intended to be tailored to the employer's needs and offered to staff. The employer would not pay any of the premiums; these would be paid for by the employees.

Long-term care insurance as a life assurance rider

Commercial Union launched the first UK product of this type in June 1991. 'Life Plus' gives an accelerated death benefit triggered by failing four out of six ADL conditions. The accelerated benefits are payable over a 50-month period, with each payment equal to 2 per cent of the sum insured. If the policyholder dies the balance of the monthly instalments is paid.

There also exist riders to dread disease insurance which pay a single lump sum benefit on failing four out of six ADLs.

Annuity and pseudo-annuity products

Enhanced annuities can provide an attractive means of financing care services for individuals who have already experienced a health breakdown and need additional income immediately. By taking account of reduced life expectancy, the level of income can be much higher than for a standard age-related annuity plan. Enhanced (or impaired life) annuities have been available for many years but have not been specifically packaged for the elderly care market. The income from these products lasts the rest of the individual's life, regardless of how long this is.

Eagle Star launched the first specifically packaged annuity product in March 1991 with its 'Care Fees Payment Plan'. It is in fact a 'pseudo-annuity' product, in that the lump sum paid by the individual is used to purchase a series of endowment policies (rather than an annuity income) which mature at regular intervals in order to pay care fees. In some cases it may be possible to agree with the care home a level of fees which is guaranteed for life. For basic-rate taxpayers,

Eagle Star pays the tax due on payments. The lump sum price depends on life expectancy, assessed within one of five risk groups. The Care Fees Payment Plan is aimed at the 'crisis' market of people who need to enter a care home immediately or who are already resident in a care home. Purchase will usually be financed through disposal of a house or other assets.

Commercial Union's 'Continuing Care Plan' is aimed at the same crisis or immediate market. It takes the form of a true rather than a pseudo annuity. That part of annuity income which does not involve capital repayment is taxable in the hands of the annuitant, though tax could possibly be avoided if the money were paid direct to a provider of care services, in the same way that long-term care insurance benefits may be tax-free if paid direct to care providers. The Inland Revenue has not confirmed that it may be possible to escape tax in this way, and has been unwilling to make a general ruling.

Equity release products

Under traditional mortgage annuity loans (home income plans), an interest-only mortgage is raised on the elderly person's property and an annuity purchased with the capital. Above a certain age the annuity income is sufficiently in excess of the mortgage interest to provide the elderly person with an additional income. Enhanced annuities which take account of the reduced life expectancy of elderly people who have already suffered a health breakdown can make the income from such equity release products more attractive at any age, but no product specifically packaged for paying care expenses has yet emerged. The net income that can be achieved by home income plans is enhanced by mortgage tax relief, but this is limited to the first £30,000 of the mortgage loan. As a result many elderly people find that home income plans are not attractive. More income can be raised through home reversion schemes, where part or all of the home is sold in return for an income and the right to occupy for life. Parting with ownership is, however, a psychological barrier.

Though equity release schemes have been available for more than 20 years, the number sold remains small in comparison with the number of elderly owner-occupied households. Hamnett (1992) has estimated that the number of clients grew from 1,850 in 1980 to just below 5,000 in 1988. There was then a more rapid expansion to 15,500 in 1989, followed by a slump back to 3,600 in 1990 as a result of the depression in the housing market and high mortgage interest rates. Equity release schemes gained a bad reputation at this time because of the sale of inappropriate products where income bonds were substituted for an annuity. The annuitant's income depended on the income bonds generating more money than the interest paid out to service the mortgage loan. With rising interest rates and falling income from the stock market-based income bonds, many elderly people found themselves facing a mounting mortgage debt and even the possibility of repossession. It is now widely accepted that only low- or zero-risk mortgage annuity or reversion schemes should be marketed, but it may take some time for elderly purchasers to regain confidence in the fundamentally sound principle of equity release.

▪ The future of financial products for long-term care

Much of the basic research that took place while these long-term care funding products were being developed was undertaken by reinsurance companies. The position reinsurers occupy in the British financial services sector is an interesting one. Insurance companies themselves have tended in recent years to focus their attention on long-term management of investment funds and offering basic protection products. The reinsurers earn their revenue from protection products and have an interest in encouraging insurance companies to develop and market new types of protection product such as long-term care insurance. Because these products are new, a share of the business is passed on to reinsurers, and this increases their revenue.

Early results of attitude surveys sponsored by reinsurers indicated that financial products for long-term care funding would appeal to a significant but minority market.

A survey sponsored by NRG Victory Reinsurance found that 17 per cent of people aged 40–70 consider it important to have long-term care insurance cover – about the same as for private medical insurance but well below the corresponding figure for pensions (66 per cent) and life assurance (62 per cent).

A survey sponsored by Swiss Re found that a rather higher proportion of their sample (of people aged 15–75) said they would 'like the option' of long-term care insurance. But these were concentrated in younger age groups; when the under-45s are excluded the Swiss Re figures are comparable with Victory's, with 18 per cent of people aged 45–64 and 9 per cent of those over 65 who would 'like the option' of long-term care insurance.

One important finding of a survey of people aged 40–70 carried out by Mercantile and General Reinsurance was that long-term care insurance is very price-sensitive. Penetration in Britain may depend on insurers devising products which meet needs economically. The German experience of long-term care insurance illustrates the point. The comprehensive but very expensive plan devised by an insurance industry committee at the instigation of government failed to attract significant numbers of purchasers.

The NRG Victory survey also investigated attitudes towards long-term care insurance as an employee benefit. The results suggest that the 'group' market will be slower to develop than the individual market, as in the United States. When interest in different employee benefits was ranked, pensions and life assurance came first, followed by permanent health insurance and private medical insurance, with long-term care insurance a long way behind.

Swiss Re asked about equity release mechanisms and found a greater interest in those than in long-term care insurance among the 45 plus age group. Twenty-three per cent of people aged 45–64 said they would 'use the capital in their house to finance private care' and 15 per cent of people aged 65 plus.

It has been argued by Munich Re that financial products for long-term care funding can best be marketed as part of a pension package. This would then ensure that the pension message promoted to people throughout their working lives also covered the possible need for care in old age.

The concept of age- or dependency-related enhancements to personal or occupational pensions has, however, received a setback with the withdrawal of Inland Revenue approval of Cannon Lincoln's

Oasis Plus plan. The case for reversing this decision is considered in Chapter 7.

Some two years after the first British long-term care funding products were launched, the consensus that has been reached within the financial services sector is as follows:

- Initial sales have been slow, despite considerable consumer interest in the idea. Reluctance to buy may have been accentuated by the recession during this period.

- Non-affordability and lack of awareness of risk are the major barriers to sales. The financial services sector faces a major task in educating the public about the importance of making private financing arrangements.

- A number of anomalies in the tax treatment of long-term care funding products need to be resolved and, more broadly, the whole issue of the relationship between long-term care funding products and the state funding system needs to be addressed.

- The market for immediate care products such as enhanced annuities is likely to develop more quickly than the market for prefunded products such as long-term care insurance.

The United States has the longest experience of long-term care funding products. The product range that eventually emerges in Britain will be very different, with many more equity release and enhanced annuity plans. Nevertheless, the USA offers a valuable model for how at least some aspects of the long-term care funding market may develop in the UK. This is because the incentives to make private provision against a background of means-tested state benefits are very similar. As in Britain, US citizens have to spend down their own resources before they become eligible for state assistance for long-term care outside their own homes. The difference, perhaps, is that Americans attach a greater stigma to reliance on state benefits.

The average age of individual purchasers of stand-alone long-term care insurance policies, which account for 94 per cent of all policies written in the USA, is 69. Employer-sponsored group long-term care insurance has reached a younger group with an average age of 43, but these policies make up only 5 per cent of the total. For long-term care riders to life assurance policies (1 per cent of all policies), the average age of US subscribers is 47.

One clear message from the USA, which will strike a chord with the British financial services sector, is that the market is slow to develop. Long-term insurance first evolved in the United States in 1974 but did not start to take off until the late 1980s. Even by 1991, the 1.9 million long-term care insurance policies sold represented a penetration of only 3 per cent of the population aged 65 and over and contributed just 1 per cent of nursing home revenues (Levit et al, 1991).

Consumer protection

Perhaps the most important issue raised by the US experience is consumer protection. Instances of poor policy design and unacceptable practices in claims control have damaged public confidence in the long-term care insurance sector. Federal and state bodies have responded with regulation which is both expensive and arguably overrestrictive. Moreover, the policy lapse rate can be high. The British financial services sector is aware of these potential problems, particularly in view of the marketing of inappropriate income bond equity release schemes to elderly people in Britain in the 1980s. There have already been some moves towards creating a self-regulatory structure which would aim to discourage inappropriate products and sales methods. The Association of British Insurers has now endorsed a Code of Conduct for selling. Self-regulation is in many ways preferable to unwieldy official regulatory devices, but it must of course be demonstrably effective.

Transparency of rules for triggering benefits

Another important issue is the degree of fairness and transparency with which prefunded long-term care financing plans distribute benefits amongst their subscribers. Some will receive benefits while others will not, so a visibly fair way of triggering benefits is required. The fairness of the trigger is particularly important in view of the long-term nature of the contracts and the criticisms that have been levelled against the financial services industry in the past, for example over the unfair treatment of the occupational pension rights of individuals who change jobs.

To date, all but one of the British providers of prefunded long-term care plans have used Activities of Daily Living (ADLs) as the trigger for receipt of benefits, borrowing from systems initially developed in the United States. ADL criteria typically include such activities as mobility, personal hygiene and getting dressed, and access to different levels of benefit may be triggered by failing on any two, three or four out of six ADLs. Nearly all British plans include a cognitive failure trigger to allow benefits to be paid to people with Alzheimer's disease or other organic causes of dementia.

The advantage of ADLs is that they are reasonably objective and transparent. ADLs can also be used to grade disability. The main alternative trigger is receipt of services, which also scores high on objectivity and transparency. However, as Berthoud (1988) points out in another context, a benefit which is paid only if outside care services are used might have an artificial influence on the balance of care. It might, for example, cause relatives to reduce their care contribution. It might also inhibit innovation in the delivery of care services, or encourage institutional care rather than home care, as did early long-term care policies in the USA which used prior treatment in hospital as a trigger.

The disadvantage of ADLs is poor targeting. A fundamental problem is that any two frail elderly people may need a widely differing level of resources to enable them to cope with an apparently identical set of problems. If standardised tests are used to determine financial entitlements according to predetermined rules, this will inevitably lead to some people receiving insufficient to cope with their problems and some people receiving far too much. Those that receive more than they 'need' will have every incentive to spend up to the limit of their entitlement while those that cannot cope with the standard entitlement are likely to place strong pressure on the funding agency for higher entitlements in order, for example, to avoid admission to a care home. Thus the ADL model for triggering access to benefits has an in-built tendency towards inefficiency (failure to match resources to needs) and inflation. A variety of mechanisms can be used to limit the inflationary tendency, but it cannot be entirely eradicated.

In effect, providers of private long-term care funding products have taken a decision that an objective method of distributing benefits is vital, even if benefits do not always match needs, because few individuals would buy their products without the assurance of objectivity and transparency.

On balance, therefore, the use of ADLs by the British financial services sector seems the appropriate option, though it does imply that private care funded by third-party payers will have a stronger tendency towards inflation than state-funded long-term care programmes.

BRITSMOs

Another approach to private funding of long-term care, though one that at present exists only as an academic proposal, is to create a private risk-sharing scheme offering comprehensive managed care services to its subscribers. Davies and Goddard (1987), at the Personal Social Services Research Unit at the University of Kent, have proposed a model for social care (long-term care) which would serve both a state-funded and a privately funded clientele, making use of experience derived from the Kent Community Care Project. The BRITSMO (British Social Care Maintenance Organisation) would offer managed social care on a pre-paid basis similar in principle to Health Maintenance Organisations (HMOs) operating in the acute health care sector in the United States. BRITSMOs might carry out the full range of managed care from financing to arranging care services by assembling packages of care from various providers. Or they might provide a brokerage service only, advising clients on the care options available.

The theoretical merit of managed social care, like managed health care, lies in the balance of incentives. BRITSMOs would have the incentive to control costs (using the same methods of rationing access to care as are currently used by social service departments), but they would also have the incentive to maintain consumer satisfaction in order to keep their enrolees from switching membership to another social care maintenance organisation.

The concepts embodied in BRITSMOs influenced the White Paper *Caring for People,* but the BRITSMO is essentially a social insurance concept and, in so far as BRITSMOs seek to serve a state-funded clientele, the concept lies uneasily alongside the means-testing of eligibility for long-term care services which is at the heart of current state funding arrangements.

5 The international context

It is only fairly recently that comparative studies of long-term care financing in different countries have started to enter the literature. The first significant contribution came from Pamela Doty (1988). Though based on data largely from the beginning of the 1980s, it still offers an excellent overview of the various models of financing which different countries have adopted, and many of the conclusions remain highly relevant to today's debate.

Doty concludes, for example, that the two key factors which tend to lead to low institutionalisation rates (low numbers of people receiving long-term care outside their own homes) are means-testing and rigorous controls on the supply of places in institutional settings. Up to the 1980s, Britain had both. During the 1980s, when the Income Support system was operating, controls on supply were effectively relaxed and institutionalisation rates increased significantly, though rigorous means-testing continued to exert a restrictive influence.

Another important conclusion drawn by Doty was that high rates of long-term care outside people's own homes appear to go hand in hand with high levels of care for people living in their own homes. At the level of international comparisons at least, long-term care outside people's own homes and care services for people living in their own homes do not appear to substitute for each other. Rather, generous access to *both* forms of care appears to reflect a high level of political commitment to the care of elderly people in general, for example in Scandinavia and the Netherlands.

A more recent paper by Joshua Weiner (1992a) looks at the present and potential contribution of private sector initiatives in financing long-term care in OECD countries. Because long-term care insurance and other private funding mechanisms at present play such a small role, Weiner concludes that more people could undoubtedly make use of these instruments. But his broad conclusion, based among other things on the affordability of private funding products, is that it is probably not realistic to envisage private schemes covering a large proportion of the population or private schemes supplanting public spending. The main justification for private sector initiatives, according to Weiner, is not so much to provide a solution to a public funding 'problem' as to improve the quality of life of the minority of people who can afford them.

The principal question addressed in this chapter is how the UK's system of state funding of long-term care compares with that in other advanced industrialised countries. To what extent is the financial risk covered by the state in other countries and to what extent do governments leave the risk with individuals, as does the British government, with those who come to need long-term care outside their own homes finding the bulk of their income and wealth absorbed in paying for it?

Brief summaries of the state financing systems in a number of OECD countries are set out in the Appendix. Though the list of countries surveyed is not exhaustive, it illustrates the range of systems that have been adopted and indicates the options open to the UK.

The summaries in the Appendix are mainly concerned with locating each country's state funding system on the continuum of universality–selectivity. At the universal end of the continuum, the social insurance principle applies and all insured individuals have a right to have their long-term care paid for by the state or the social insurance agency regardless of income or assets. At the selective end of the continuum, the welfare principle applies and state funding is restricted to those individuals who have no resources of their own.

The Appendix focuses principally on state financing of long-term care outside people's own homes rather than care services for people living in their own homes, first because information is more readily available and the means-testing rules are much more clearly set at national level, and second because care outside people's own homes accounts for the bulk of state funding – typically about 70–75 per cent in those countries for which information is available.

It should be noted that none of the countries surveyed, even those whose state funding system is the most generous, give people who need long-term care the same degree of financial protection as patients receiving treatment for acute illness. Thus, while in most countries no co-payment, or only a small one, is required for acute hospital treatment, all the countries surveyed without exception require long-term residents to make a substantial financial contribution to the cost of state-funded long-term care outside people's own homes. All the advanced industrialised countries surveyed provide at least a minimum safety net of state cover for those who need care but who have no resources of their own.

▪ Different models of state funding for care outside people's own homes

The various systems of state funding of long-term care outside people's own homes found in the survey of OECD countries have been classified into five types.

1 Social insurance entitlement: No resident charges

No country surveyed meets these criteria.

2 Social insurance entitlement: Flat-rate charges

Canada is the only one of the countries surveyed where this mode of state financing applies to all long-term care outside people's own homes. The entire population of Canada is covered by a state insurance scheme for long-term care outside people's own homes on a non-means-tested basis. Residents are, however, liable for a charge (or co-payment) which is intended to go towards the board and housing element of cost. The co-payment varies from province to province but is typically about $750 to $800 per month for a shared room (1992 figures). As the minimum pensioner income by comparison is about $900 per month, this leaves the poorest individuals in long-term care outside their own homes with some income for personal expenses. No claim is made on the individual's other private income or assets.

For a single room, however, the charge is typically $1,700 per month. Though the Canadian system of funding achieves the objective of preventing impoverishment of long-term care residents who would have to spend down their resources under a means-testing regime, it does not assure equality of access and does not allow a full range of choice of amenity for less well-off people. Individuals without means apart from the basic state pension are unable to afford a single room.

In some other countries, only part of long-term care provision outside people's own homes can be classed as an insured entitlement. The UK offers the best example, where a diminishing minority (12 per cent in 1992) of frail elderly people in long-term care outside their own homes are resident in NHS long-stay hospitals and wards and have no obligation to pay other than losing Attendance Allowance and having their state pension reduced to a 'pocket money' level. The NHS makes no claim on long-stay patients' other income or on their assets – in contrast with the rigorous income and assets means test applied to elderly people receiving state-funded long-term care in non-NHS settings in the UK. Germany is another country where a minority of frail elderly people receive 'free' long-term care outside their own homes, though in this case it arises from unintended use of acute care hospital beds for long-term care (Doty, 1988).

3 Social insurance for the care element – Welfare benefit for hotel costs

This is the model which has been adopted in France, where individuals in long-term care outside their own homes have a non-means-tested entitlement to part payment from health insurance funds (*assurance maladie*), which is intended to contribute to the care element of costs. State payment for the hotel element of the costs of long-term care outside people's own homes, on the other hand, is made via the social security system at municipal level (*aide sociale*) and is subject to a severe means test, which takes both income and assets into account and requires individuals to spend down all their assets and income before becoming eligible.

The non-means-tested health insurance fund contribution is graded according to the type of care facility. At the beginning of 1993, the national schedule provided FF202.20 per day towards the cost of care in a long-stay hospital, FF124.90 per day for care in a care home with nursing care (roughly corresponding to a UK nursing home), and FF16.40 per day for care in a care home without nursing care (the rough equivalent of a UK residential home).

Recently the German government, which has hitherto applied one of the most severe means-testing regimes of any OECD country, decided to adopt a partial social insurance model similar to the French one for funding long-term care outside people's own homes. Towards the end of 1992 the German legislature agreed in principle to the creation of a new funding system by January 1996. A non-means-tested entitlement to long-term care benefits will be added to the statutory health insurance fund. In the case of long-term care outside people's own homes, the new state benefit is intended, as in France, to cover the care element of costs only. The nursing home benefit has been set at DM2,100 per month (or the equivalent when implemented), which will cover rather more than half the typical nursing home charge of DM3,500–4,000 per month. A severe means-testing regime will continue to apply to the hotel element of charges for long-term care outside people's own homes. It has been agreed that the cost of state long-term care insurance (which is expected to amount to 1.7 per cent of payroll initially, compared with 8–12 per cent of payroll for acute health care) will be paid half by employers' contributions and half by employees' contributions. The only outstanding issue is how employers are to be compensated. German employers have argued that they have the highest payroll overheads in Europe already. One proposal is to pay for the cost of the new benefit by reducing employee entitlements to sick pay for the first few days of sickness. Another is to reduce holiday entitlement.

4 Income-tested welfare benefit

For those countries which apply the welfare principle to state funding of both the care and hotel elements of long-term care outside people's own homes, the least severe form of means-testing takes into account only the individual's income – not assets – in determining entitlement to state benefits. Sweden comes nearest to this model. Individuals receiving state-funded long-term care in nursing homes pay a variable charge which is equal to their social security pension plus a percentage of their other income, which varies locally but is typically 60–80 per cent. Elderly people in Sweden used to receive the first year of long-term care outside their own homes free of charge, but this was discontinued in 1991 as an economy measure. For most people there is no assets test, though assets are taken into account in determining charges for state-funded long-term care outside people's own homes if they are in excess of the federal wealth tax threshold. For this minority, the value of an individual's owner-occupied home is taken into account when determining charges, though only the taxation value, which is much less than the open market value.

5 Income- and asset-tested welfare benefit

This is the model which has been adopted by the UK, the United States, to a large extent the Netherlands and, until the recent policy change described above is implemented, Germany.

At its most severe, means-testing for eligibility for state benefits to pay for long-term care outside people's own homes has the following features:

- Both income and assets are taken into account, including the value of any property owned by the individual entering care.

- There is no upper limit on the contribution individuals are expected to make from their personal resources.

- A charge is placed on any non-liquid assets so that the state can recover any sums due under the means-testing rules when the assets have been disposed of.

- There are strictly applied rules to prevent divestment of assets or other means of circumventing the means test.

The existing German system is possibly the most draconian. Income and assets must be spent down before an individual qualifies for benefits from the German equivalent of Income Support, the asset threshold of DM4,500 is lower than the UK threshold of £8,000, there is no parallel 'free' provision under the health care system except for some unintended use of acute hospitals, the state recovers any sums owing after disposal of assets, and the authorities have a claim on assets that the elderly person has given away up to ten years previously. The state can also seek a (small) contribution from the sons of the elderly person – though not their daughters.

The United States means test is the next most severe of the systems surveyed. Here, too, parallel 'free' provision of long-term care outside people's own homes is very limited. Medicare, the non-means-tested federal insurance programme, pays for less than 3 per cent of all the costs of long-term care outside people's own homes. The main source of state funding is Medicaid, the state welfare system, for which eligibility depends on all other income and assets having been exhausted. Impoverishment prior to receipt of benefits is viewed as a particularly harsh condition in the United States because of the stigma attached to dependence on welfare programmes. There is a 30-month rule on divestment of assets, which is less restrictive than the present German ten-year rule. The USA means test is also less severe in its treatment of owner-occupied property. Medicaid may subject property to a lien and seek reimbursement when it is finally sold, but it does not always do so.

The Netherlands is another country with severe means-testing for state-funded long-term care outside people's own homes. As in the United States, a small amount of such care is funded through the health insurance system – about 6,000 nursing home places funded through the Exceptional Medical Expenses Scheme (AWBZ). When the AWBZ was introduced in the 1970s nursing home care was free, but a personal contribution was introduced in the early 1980s as an economy measure. This personal contribution is income-tested but not asset-tested and is capped at a limit of 2,000 guilder per month. The great bulk of long-term care provision outside people's own homes in the Netherlands, however, is not in nursing homes but in homes for the aged, with about 130,000 places, for which the means test is much more severe. Access to state funding for homes for the aged is both income- and asset-tested, and the value of any owner-occupied home is taken into account. Under the Dekker reforms, homes for the aged may in the future be brought within a new basic health insurance scheme. The effect of this may, however, be to increase the severity of the means test for long-term care outside people's own homes overall, since the proposal is that the severe means test which now applies to homes for the aged should also apply to nursing homes under the new basic health insurance scheme.

As in the United States, Germany and the Netherlands, state funding of long-term care in the UK is subject to an income and assets means test which includes the value of owner-occupied homes and any other assets, the total value of which is above £8,000. However, the UK means test has operated less rigidly – at least up to April 1993 – than the German or US systems, first because of the coexistence of non-means-tested NHS long-stay provision for a significant though diminishing proportion of people entering long-term care outside their own homes, and, second, because the Income Support rules have allowed owner-occupiers who have taken steps to sell their property to remain eligible for Income Support in independent sector care homes for six months and sometimes longer. The crucially important feature of this rule, which became widely used with the depression in the housing market, was that DSS offices did not place a charge on claimants' property and did not seek to recover the cost of the first 6–12 months' care from the claimant after the property had been sold. From April 1993, however, the situation has changed. The care element of state funding of long-term care has passed to local authorities, who are empowered to place a charge on claimants' property and to obtain reimbursement after the sale. Thus, while owner-occupiers who are unable to sell their property will still be able to claim Income Support under the new system (depending on their other income and assets) to cover the 'hotel' element of care home costs, they will no longer be able to do so without having to pay back to the local authority, on eventual disposal of the asset, all that they owe for the period prior to the sale of the property. This represents a significant tightening of the UK means test from April 1993.

Family contributions

In both France and Germany, the state may seek a small contribution from the children of elderly people receiving state-funded long-term care outside their own homes. The only country surveyed where children are liable to pay the full cost of their elderly parents' care is Switzerland. It has been known for middle-aged Swiss people who have lost all contact with their parents to be presented with a bill for nursing home care after the elderly parent's death. Swiss children's liability has, however, to be understood in the context of Swiss law, which does not allow parents to disinherit their children. In any case, Swiss children can avoid payment by repudiating their inheritance. In practice, therefore, the position in Switzerland amounts to something very similar to that in the UK, where children 'pay' for the care of their parents out of their inheritance.

■ Conclusions on the different models of state funding for care outside people's own homes

Although the Canadian model of social insurance with co-payments has a different point of departure from the French model of partial social insurance, these two systems (and in due course the German model as well) display a high degree of convergence. In practice, all three provide non-means-tested state benefits for the *care* element of long-term care outside people's own homes, while the individual pays the *hotel* costs, with a welfare safety net for those who cannot.

In essence, a simplified classification of state funding of long-term care outside people's own homes would contrast the Canadian, French and new German social insurance models with the welfare model exemplified by the old German system, the USA, the Netherlands, the UK and even Sweden.

Changes in state funding regimes in recent years have not all been in the same direction. The German decision to opt for partial social insurance to cover the care element of long-term care outside people's own homes is the single most important recent change. It represents a major extension of state-funded entitlements. But other countries have taken steps in the opposite direction and have restricted entitlements on economy grounds. Examples include Sweden, which has discontinued the previous entitlement to a year of non-means-tested nursing home care, the Netherlands, which is considering applying a more severe means-testing regime to nursing home care, and the UK, where the effect of the state funding changes introduced in April 1993 has been to make the asset test more extensively applied to new care home entrants.

Comparative institutionalisation rates

Numbers of care home places, where available, are set out in the country summaries in the Appendix. The main purpose of these statistics is to indicate where the bulk of long-term care outside people's own homes is provided, in those cases where means-testing rules vary within a country according to the type of care facility. The statistics are not, however, sufficiently reliable to allow an international comparison of institutionalisation rates. The reasons why no such comparison has been attempted are:

- Variations in the age mix of elderly populations in different countries can make simple comparisons misleading.

- There can be significant hidden use of acute hospital beds for long-term care, leading to underestimation of the total provision of care outside people's own homes (for example Germany and Switzerland).

- Lack of good data on some facilities can also lead to underestimation (for example 'board and care' homes in the United States).

- There is a lack of clarity over whether certain facilities should be included as institutions (for example conversion of many Swedish nursing homes into blocks of service flats for elderly people).

- There are special, time-limited reasons for differences in institutionalisation, for example very high non-marriage rates among Swedish women born in the first decade of the century.

Bearing these caveats in mind, the UK remains at the low end of the range of institutionalisation rates among OECD countries, despite the significant increase in age-specific utilisation of care homes which took place in the 1980s when Income Support funding became freely available (see pp 25–30). In Doty's (1988) international survey of long-term care, she found that Canada, Sweden, Switzerland and the

Netherlands were at the higher end of the range and Germany, with its hidden use of acute hospitals for long-term care, was at the bottom. Though the UK was not included in the study, its rate of institutionalisation would have been close to the lower end of the OECD range.

■ International comparisons of state funding for care for people living in their own homes

Information is much less readily available for long-term care services for people living in their own homes than for care outside people's own homes, and this makes international comparisons more difficult. Whereas rules governing charges and means-testing for care outside people's own homes are typically set at national level, the rules governing charges for care for people living in their own homes are typically subject to local discretion.

One of the few generalisations that can be made is that health-related services such as qualified nurse visits to people in their own homes and day care provided in a medical setting tend to be funded by the state on an insured entitlement basis rather than a welfare basis, either free of charge or subject to small, non-income-related charges. Non-health-related domiciliary care services, on the other hand, with no medical or qualified nursing input, are more likely to be provided on a welfare basis with more frequent use of income-related charges. The often arbitrary division in the UK between NHS 'health' services and local authority 'social' services is mirrored in other countries under their particular administrative arrangements.

In the UK, the main state-funded, long-term 'health' service for people living in their own homes is district nursing and the main domiciliary 'social' service is the provision of home helps/home care workers. District nursing is not subject to charges. The government's position with regard to home helps/home care workers and other local authority services for people living in their own homes is that local authorities should seek to recover the full economic cost of providing day and domiciliary services wherever this can be done without causing hardship to the user. Local authorities have the discretion to formulate their own charging policies, however, and these vary widely from quite substantial income-related charges to small flat-rate charges to, sometimes, free provision.

Although it has not been possible, in the research carried out for this book, to compare the volumes of state resources devoted to long-term care for people living in their own homes in different countries, as far as the broad division of responsibility between the state and the individual is concerned the UK is squarely located in the European mainstream. Among the larger European Community countries, France and Germany apply what amount to very similar funding principles, with free home nursing services and home help/home care services subject to income-tested charges. In a number of other countries, means-testing is somewhat more severe than in the UK, with charges for home nursing services as well.

A further generalisation that can be made is that, whereas income-related charges are frequently levied, none of the countries surveyed takes assets into account when setting charges for state-funded 'health' or 'social' long-term care services.

■ International comparisons of state funding for carers

A recently published research paper commissioned by the Social Security Advisory Committee (Glendinning and McLaughlin, 1993) gives the results of a comparison of state funding for unpaid carers in seven European countries: Finland, France, Germany, Ireland, Italy, Sweden and the UK. The authors conclude that current levels of financial support for unpaid carers are low in the UK compared with most of the other European countries studied. A positive aspect of UK policy, however, which is not seen elsewhere, is the UK's recognition through the Invalid Care Allowance that carers should be supported in their own right – rather than through people needing care or as substitutes for statutory agencies which would otherwise have to provide care.

6 How big is the demographic time bomb?

We know that long-term care is going to cost more in the future than it does now. But how much more will it cost? And is there any justification for some of the more alarmist scenarios of the burden of care escalating beyond control and becoming 'unaffordable' in the future unless new sources of non-state finance can be tapped. There are numerous academic studies which have projected total health care costs for the elderly population, but it is only very recently that attempts have been made to separate out long-term care costs (Robins and Wittenberg, 1992). The conclusion reached below is that extrapolation of *known* trends does not support the view that long-term care is beyond the bounds of affordability on current financing arrangements, though it is of course possible that the alarmist scenario might prove accurate – for example, if as yet unknown advances in medical technology serve to extend life expectation significantly without reducing disability, or if carers start to withdraw their unpaid labour en masse.

The best estimate, based on the Government Actuary's principal population projection and assuming constant age-specific usage of long-term care services, is that the proportion of GDP spent on the long-term care of elderly people would have to rise from 1.5 per cent in 1992 to 3.5 per cent by the time demand peaks in the year 2051 in order to maintain services at today's level and standards. If 70 per cent of this continues to be publicly funded, the state would find its financial commitment to the long-term care of elderly people rising from a little over 1 per cent of GDP in 1992 to 2.5 per cent in 2051. These are large amounts of money by anyone's standards, and they may seem daunting in the context of short-term imperatives to contain Britain's public sector borrowing requirement. But in the very long term, encompassing a number of economic cycles, it would be absurd to conclude on present evidence that the state must seek alternative funding arrangements because it cannot afford to pay for the care required. Whether the state can afford to pay for long-term care is a political question, the answer to which is in no way pre-empted by economics.

Assuring the availability of sufficient public and private resources to pay for long-term care in the future is a major challenge, but it would be wholly misleading to represent it as an impending crisis requiring a major adjustment in the economy. Funding long-term care is a pressing issue not so much because of the macro-economic implications, but because of the difficult and sometimes traumatic consequences for individuals and families if finance for the right sort of provision is not available at the right time. It also needs to be recognised that Britain's demographic 'problems' are less severe than those of some other countries such as Germany and Japan, where the effects of a low birth rate (Germany) and low mortality rates (Japan) mean there will be a greater concentration than in Britain of people at the very top of the age distribution (OECD, 1988b).

▬ Demographic trends

Though, as stressed above, future demand for long-term care resources cannot be characterised as 'unaffordable' under existing financing arrangements, the Government Actuary's most recent national population projections undoubtedly lend support to the alarmist school (OPCS, 1993). The principal projection, based on 1991 census data, has made a downward revision in assumed mortality rates for elderly age groups, with a consequent substantial increase in the projected number of survivors in the older age groups most at risk of needing long-term care services (see *Figure 4*).

Figure 4 indicates that the number of people aged 85 and over in the UK is set to rise from 897,000 in 1991 to 1,202,000 in 2001 and 3,105,000 at its peak in 2051. It may be even higher if death rates continue to decline more rapidly than the OPCS principal projections assume. Grundy (1992) has pointed out that mortality forecasts in the

Figure 4 United Kingdom elderly population, 1991–2061, principal projection

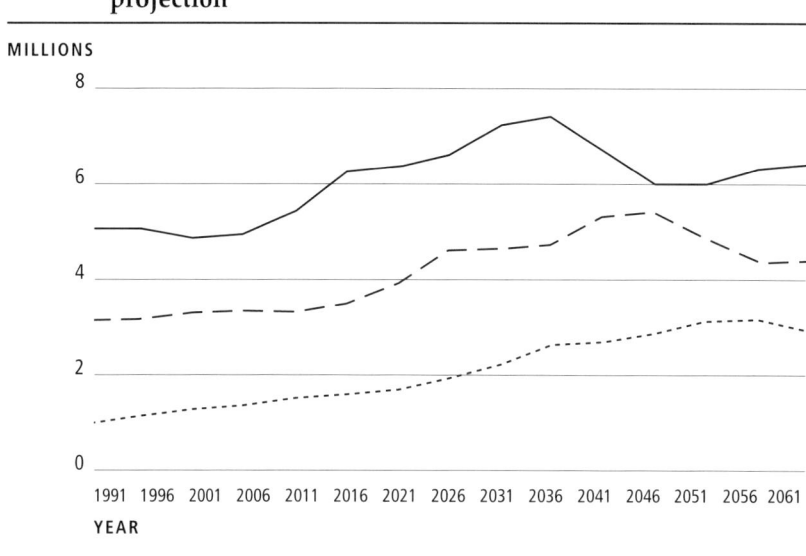

Source: Government Actuary's Department, unpublished. (Projections for England and Wales by age are published in OPCS Monitor PP2 93/1.)

past have consistently underestimated the decline in death rates at older ages.

Another important demographic trend, itself a consequence of the growing numbers of very old people, is an increase in the proportion of elderly people living alone. Forty-seven per cent of individuals aged 75 or over lived alone in 1990, compared with 45 per cent in 1991 and 35 per cent in 1971 (Grundy, 1992). Part of the change is due to a decline in the extent of co-residence of elderly people and their younger relatives. According to Wall (1984), for example, 25 per cent of elderly widows lived with an ever-married child in 1962, compared with 10 per cent in 1990. The trend towards solitary living is expected to continue: the Department of the Environment projects a net increase of over 600,000 elderly single-person households in Britain between 1986 and 2001. On the face of it, this trend has major implications for the funding of long-term care because living alone is the largest demographic risk factor – after age itself – for entry into care in NHS or care home settings. To the extent, however, that elderly people are now choosing to live alone – whereas previously people may have been constrained to live with relatives for reasons of economy and housing supply – there is no necessarily constant relationship between living alone and risk of needing long-term care.

▬ Age-specific usage of long-term care services

Because rates of disability and dependence escalate so rapidly with increasing old age (*Tables 12* and *13* and *Figure 5*), it is the growing numbers of very old people that will fuel the demand for long-term care services in the future. Demand for care in NHS or care home settings, the most expensive form of long-term care, escalates rapidly with age. Some 1 per cent of the population aged 65–74 live in some form of institutional setting, whether an NHS hospital, a local authority residential home, or a private or voluntary residential or nursing home. For people aged 85 and over, the proportion is estimated to reach 29 per

Table 12 Risk of living in a long-stay hospital or care home by age, England, 1991

	<65	65–74	75–84	85+
% Living in homes or hospitals*	0.05	1.1	6.7	28.8

* Includes people in residential and nursing homes, NHS long-stay geriatric hospitals and wards for elderly severely mentally ill people.

Source: Laing and Buisson, 1993a.

Table 13 Age-specific usage of certain community care services, Great Britain, 1986

	65–69	70–74	75–79	80–84	85+	65+
% Visited by home help in previous month	1	5	11	22	36	9
% Visited by district nurse in previous month	2	2	5	10	20	5
% Receiving meals on wheels in previous month	0	1	3	6	11	2

Source: General Household Survey, 1986.

Figure 5 Estimates of prevalence of disability among adults in Great Britain by age and severity* category

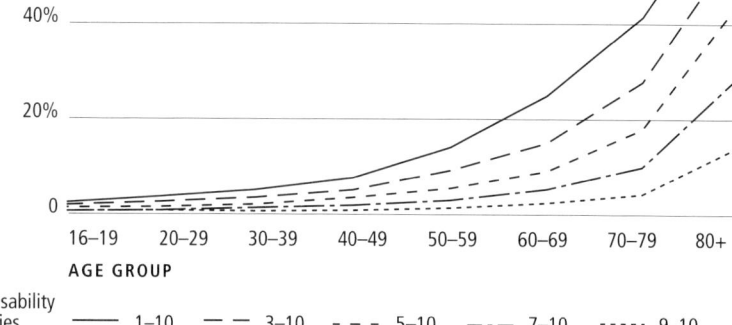

PERCENTAGE OF
POPULATION

AGE GROUP

OPCS Disability Categories   —— 1–10   — — 3–10   - - - 5–10   —·— 7–10   ····· 9–10

*Category 1 least severe disability, category 10 most severe disability.

Source: OPCS surveys of disability in Great Britain (Martin et al, 1988).

cent. This steep gradient means that, other things being equal, another 77,000 places in long-stay hospitals or care homes will be needed in the UK between 1992 and the year 2000 in order to keep pace with demographic pressures, taking the number of such places in the UK to 623,000. Looking forward as far as 2051, on the heroic assumptions that population projections will prove accurate and age-specific rates of institutionalisation will remain constant, the number of places in long-stay hospitals and care homes can be projected to reach 1,290,000.

▬ Projections of the cost of long-term care

How reliable are these projections? The method used here is to take age-specific usage rates for care in NHS or care home settings (see

Table 12) as a proxy for usage of care in NHS or care home settings and care for people living in their own homes combined, and apply these to official population projections. The resulting 'best estimate', making no allowance for rising expectations, for any price increases above the general rate of inflation, or for any other long-term change that might affect the cost of care, is that the volume of resources devoted to long-term care in the UK would have to grow by 136 per cent between 1991 and 2051 (the year of peak demand) in order to keep pace with additional care needs arising from the ageing of the population alone (see *Figure 6*).

The percentage increase in resources required for long-term care is much greater than that for acute health care services. Similar estimates by the same author (ABPI, 1991), updated in the light of the latest

Figure 6 Long-term care resources required to keep pace with demographic change in the UK (Index 1991 = 100)

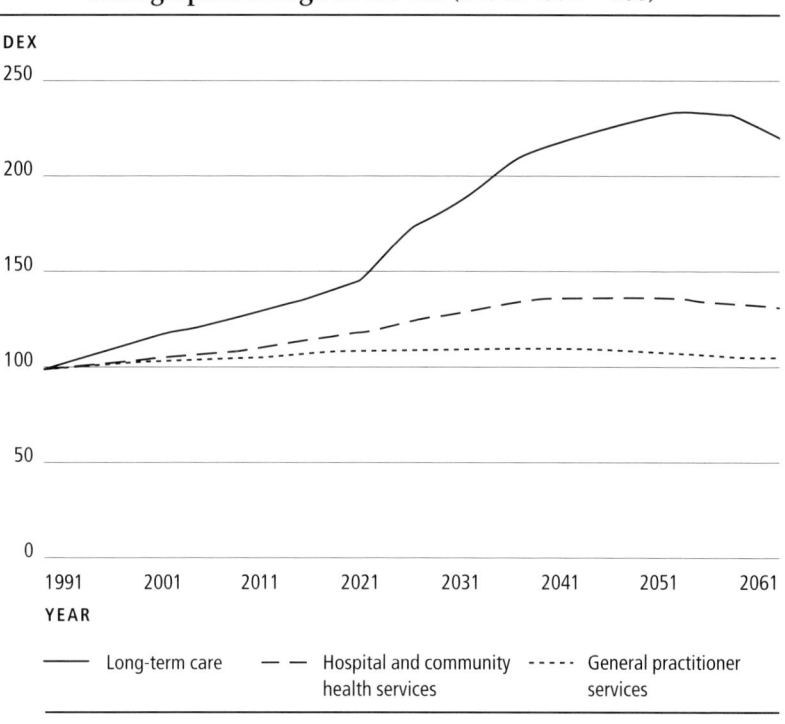

population projections, indicate a 37 per cent additional resource requirement for NHS hospital and community health services and a 6 per cent additional resource requirement for general practitioner services by 2051.

The assumption behind the projections is that all other things apart from demographic change will remain equal. It would be truly remarkable if that were the case, though it is possible that the other things which affect the future cost of long-term care will cancel each other out. The following subsections look in detail at the three major factors which could lead the 'best estimate' of future long-term care costs to be seriously wrong. These are: future changes in mortality/ morbidity rates in old age, people's willingness to care for their relatives, and the rate of inflation in the cost of care.

Mortality and morbidity in old age

Medical technology is the wild card in any future projection of long-term care costs. The most pessimistic scenario for the future might involve advances in medical technology which bring about a greatly increased expectation of life but without any corresponding reduction in morbidity from age-related conditions which are not immediately life-threatening, such as arthritis, dementia and depression. Ultimately, in such a 'domesday' scenario, the resulting burden of care might only be contained by withdrawing from old people the right to medical treatment (within available resources) which is enshrined in the NHS Act of 1948. An 'optimistic' scenario, on the other hand, might envisage the major degenerative diseases of old age being conquered and most people living active lives until shortly before their deaths.

An international debate has developed over the last 10–15 years on the relationship between changes in mortality and morbidity, triggered by the unexpectedly large decreases in mortality among older people that have been observed in developed countries in recent decades. While the decline in mortality is not disputed, it is not clear what has happened to morbidity and disability rates among elderly people during this time.

Fries (1980, 1989) has set out an optimistic hypothesis of the 'compression of morbidity'. He suggests that improvements in lifestyle and health care have had the effect of extending healthy life, with disability compressed into a shorter period as life expectancy reaches its hypothetical ceiling. Kramer (1980) and Gruenberg (1977), on the other hand, have presented the 'pessimistic' view that the recent fall in mortality has not been accompanied by a decrease in morbidity but is the result of an increase in life expectancy among people in poor health. Kramer thus predicts increasingly poor health in elderly populations and a consequent 'pandemic of mental disorders and associated chronic diseases'.

In fact, there is little solid evidence to support either of these polarised viewpoints. Fries cites some interesting supporting data for heart disease, but little for any other conditions. The data supporting the pessimistic scenario are similarly thin. Robine and Ritchie (1991), for example, have reviewed all studies in North America and Europe which have attempted to measure disability-free life expectancy against total life expectancy. They conclude that the ratio of disability-free to total life expectancy has decreased in both the United States (between 1970 and 1980) and England and Wales (between 1976 and 1985). This seems to support the pessimistic hypothesis, but the calculations are themselves highly suspect. They are based on a method proposed by Sullivan (1971) which uses institutionalisation rates and prevalence of long- and short-term restrictions in activity derived from national health studies. Changes in institutionalisation rates, however, are not a good proxy for disability. The increase in the rate of institutionalisation in England and Wales in the 1980s (see *Figure 2*), for example, was certainly at least in part a consequence of the ready availability of Income Support funding for independent care homes. Data from national health surveys, moreover, are subjective. In Britain, the increase over time in self-reported, limiting, long-standing illness found in successive General Household Surveys cannot seriously be taken as an objective measure of the changing level of disability in the community. As the commentary to the General Household Survey itself points out, 'It should be noted that, as these measures are based on people's subjective assessments of their health, changes over time may reflect changes in people's expectations of health as well as in the prevalence or duration of chronic sickness' (Smyth and Browne, 1992).

The conclusion to be drawn is that we do not know whether age-specific disability rates have been increasing or decreasing in the past, or whether they will increase or decrease in the future. Certainly, the evidence one way or another is not sufficiently strong to alter the way in which we should plan the funding of long-term care in future years.

Care provided by unpaid carers

Care provided by unpaid carers is the bedrock of the entire system of long-term care in Britain and all other countries. The 1985 General Household Survey for the first time provided reliable baseline data on carers in Britain. The results revealed an estimated 1,400,000 people devoting 20 hours or more to caring for elderly, sick or disabled people (Green, 1988). As already noted (see p 48), it is estimated that in the (unlikely) event that the state had entirely to replace the labour of those providing unpaid care to elderly people, the cost would amount to an annualised £32.5 billion at April 1992, dwarfing the £9.1 billion spent on formal (paid) long-term care services for elderly people. Anything that poses a threat to the supply of unpaid care therefore has potentially massive implications for the cost of formal (paid) care in future years.

The scale of care provided by unpaid carers that is revealed by the 1985 General Household Survey seems to support Parker's (1990) comment that: 'one of the most persistent misconceptions about "modern" society is that the family no longer cares for its dependants, especially the elderly'. Nevertheless, there remains considerable concern about the possible future effects of the break-up of traditional family structures and changes in working patterns among women. To what extent is this concern justified?

Divorce has been cited as a potential source of weakening of the family bonds which lead people to provide care for elderly relatives. After a sharp rise in the 1970s, the UK divorce rate reached a plateau in the 1980s, but the legacy of divorce will persist for many decades. It is possible that the more complex family ties created by divorce may lessen people's willingness to provide care. There is as yet little evidence that this is happening, but it is probably too early to say. Analysis of the 1985 General Household Survey of carers (Grundy and Harrop, 1992) indicates that there is no marked difference between married and divorced women as regards caring for elderly parents or parents-in-law. And among men aged 45–54, the incidence of caring for a parent or parent-in-law was significantly higher among divorced than among married men.

Geographical dispersal of families may also pose a threat to caring. Employment-associated migration of children to other parts of the UK and abroad may make caring more difficult to arrange and more expensive. But here again there is as yet no firm evidence to indicate that the availability of care has diminished in consequence.

The changing employment patterns of women have also been cited as a potential threat to the provision of care. According to the House of Commons Social Services Committee (HMSO, 1990a): 'Perhaps the largest single factor which may affect informal care in the future is the level of participation in the labour market.' However, it is not at all clear whether labour force participation amongst potential carers is in fact on the increase. The most recent projections from the Department of Employment (Department of Employment, 1992) are that while labour force participation is increasing among women aged below 45, the percentage of women aged 45 or over in paid employment is not expected to change significantly between now and the end of the century.

Concern about the impact of employment is not just a matter of the number of women in the labour force, but of the types of jobs they increasingly have access to and the breakdown in gender stereotypes, which may make women less likely to accept the role of unpaid carer. Here again, however, there is little evidence of any detrimental impact on the provision of care. Grundy and Harrop's (1992) analysis of the 1985 General Household Survey of carers failed to show any significant association between women's employment status and the provision of care to a co-resident elderly parent – though the results are based on small numbers. Moreover, the focus of attention on women carers ignores the contribution of men as carers. Though women are more likely to be carers than men, the difference is not substantial according to the 1985 General Household Survey results (Green, 1988).

While a number of socio-demographic trends give rise to concern about the future availability of care provided by unpaid carers, there are also some changes in the demographic pipeline which may reinforce, rather than undermine, the availability of such care. For example, fewer very old people will be never-married or childless. Timaeus (1986) has estimated that while 26 per cent of women who reached the age of 60 in 1971–76 would have no surviving children at the age of 85, among women becoming 60 during the period 1991–96 the proportion childless at 85 would be only 16 per cent.

Reviewing the evidence, Grundy (1992) concludes that there appears to be little evidence at present to support some of the more alarmist predictions about the effects of divorce and women's employment on family support for old people, though she does warn that attitudes may change, not only among carers but among elderly people themselves. Attitudinal data from Norway, for example, show a substantial shift between 1967 and 1989 in elderly people's preference for formal (public) services rather than family assistance (Daatland, 1990). In Britain it is possible that the next generation of carers and very elderly people may adopt patterns of care different from those of the current generation.

The rate of inflation in the unit cost of care

According to *Figure 6*, the volume of resources for long-term care of elderly people in the UK would have to increase by 136 per cent between 1991 and 2051 simply to keep pace with the ageing of the population. This would mean the amount of GDP devoted to the long-term care of elderly people increasing from 1.5 per cent at present to 3.5 per cent in 2051, on the assumption that the price of care rises in line with GDP per capita (that is, roughly in line with average earnings). This seems a reasonable assumption since labour accounts for the bulk of the cost of care and the opportunities for increasing the productivity of labour in long-term care must be limited.

If, however, the price of care were to rise at a rate significantly different from average earnings (or GDP per capita), the implications for the cost of long-term care by the middle of the next century could be alarming. A compound rate of growth in prices of 1 per cent higher than the average earnings index would require an upward adjustment from the projected 3.5 per cent of GDP absorbed by long-term care of elderly people in 2051 to 6.4 per cent.

Conceptually, it is necessary to distinguish between pure price inflation – that is, changes over time in the price of the same unit of service – and inflation resulting from higher rates of use of care services or from improved standards or amenities. It is not always possible to separate the two factors satisfactorily. Broadly, however, it is the latter factor, utilisation rates and service content, which has been the major source of inflation over and above the average earnings index in the past, and it is likely to remain so in the future.

As regards past experience, the evidence for this assertion includes:

- limited inflation in the fees charged by independent care homes;

- significant increases in utilisation rates for long-term care in NHS or care home settings;

- increases in state spending on long-term care for people living in their own homes well in excess of labour cost inflation.

Survey data on the fees charged by independent care homes, which now provide the bulk of long-term care outside people's own homes in the UK, are available for the period 1988–1992. Analysis by Laing and Buisson (1993a) has found that average care home fees have risen at a rate intermediate between the average earnings index and weighted average upratings in Income Support limits. The care home sector is highly price-competitive and, on this limited evidence, there appears to be no inbuilt tendency for care home fees to rise faster than average earnings.

Most of the change in the cost of long-term care in NHS or care home settings over the past decade has been due to changes in service utilisation and content, not to pure price inflation. *Figure 2* shows how the likelihood of being in long-term care in NHS or care home settings in the UK increased by 27 per cent between 1981 and 1992, after allowing for differences in the age structure of the elderly population – presumably as a result of the ready availability of Income Support funding. There was also a significant deflationary shift in the content

of care services, away from expensive long-stay hospital beds and towards less expensive private and voluntary nursing and residential
homes.

Over the last decade, usage of care services for people living in
their own homes also appears to have increased significantly. It can be
estimated from *Table 5* that real spending on local authority home
help/home care services grew by an average 4.7 per cent between
1978/79 and 1989/90. Information presented to the House of Commons Social Services Committee (HMSO, 1990b) shows that real
spending on district nursing grew even faster, at 5.7 per cent per
annum between 1977/78 and 1988/89. Since these services are almost
pure labour, and nursing and care assistant labour costs did not increase any more rapidly than earnings in general, it appears that increased volume of services has accounted for most of the increase in
spending in the past.

Future inflation in the costs of care

There is no prima facie reason for supposing that prices of inputs into
long-term care will, in the future, rise at a rate any different from general inflation. The largest element of cost will continue to be labour.
Shortages of young people entering nursing during the 1990s will
tend, other things being equal, to bid up the price of skilled nursing
staff, but the inflationary impact will be limited by the existence of a
large pool of older, qualified nurses who are not professionally active.
More generally, long-term care will absorb increasingly large numbers
of typically part-time female care assistants, but any inflationary pressures on the price of labour will be determined not so much by demand within the health care system as by demand for labour in the
economy as a whole.

It is then necessary to look at other inbuilt inflationary pressures
which may cause spending to diverge significantly from the projected
increase in the share of GDP to be absorbed by the long-term care of
elderly people from 1.5 per cent in 1992 to 3.5 per cent in 2051. These
include state regulation, rising expectations and the way in which entitlements are triggered in private insurance schemes. Countervailing

deflationary pressures will include state funding constraints and, possibly, gains in efficiency. Each of these factors is considered in turn.

REGULATION

Implementation of the 1984 Registered Homes Act led to significant increases in care home costs as increased staffing levels were required immediately and more demanding physical standards were required over time. The cost inflation brought about by the Act has now largely worked its way through the system, though some inflationary pressures do remain as regulators in health and local authorities seek, for example, to decrease the number of double and multi-occupied rooms. In the long term, the key determinant of regulatory cost push in the care home sector will be the extent to which regulators, or any new legislative provisions, continue to seek higher physical and staffing standards. Minimum physical standards in the care home sector remain fairly low, for example minimum room sizes, and there is certainly potential for further cost inflation there. In the case of staffing, however, which is the main element of cost, there is no strong reason to suppose that higher staff–resident ratios will be sought by regulators in the future.

As far as long-term care for people living in their own homes is concerned, the independent sector plays a relatively small role at present and regulation is minimal. As the scale of independent sector care for people living in their own homes increases, there will inevitably be pressure for stricter regulation and this may impose extra costs on such care.

RISING EXPECTATIONS

People aged 85 in 1993 were born in the first decade of the century and were young adults during the depression years. It is often said that their expectations are wholly different from those of the elderly generations which will follow them, especially the economically privileged baby boom generation which will reach very old age in the third decade of the twenty-first century. For those who enter long-term care in NHS or care home settings, it seems reasonable to expect that future consumers will reinforce regulators' pressures for improved physical standards and amenities and this will be a further source of cost-push inflation. On the other hand, there is no strong reason to suppose that rising expectations will lead to general increases in staff–resident ratios. Nor is there any strong reason to suppose that the baby boom generation, which was not brought up to expect personal service, will be intrinsically more demanding than the present elderly generation in respect of care for people living in their own homes.

Rules for triggering entitlements in private long-term care insurance

To the extent that private long-term care insurance schemes develop as important sources of long-term care funding in the future, they are likely to be subject to much stronger inflationary pressures than public sector budgets, particularly for care for people living in their own homes. The reason lies in the different approaches to triggering benefits.

As noted above, a fundamental problem faced by any third-party funding agency deciding how to trigger benefits is that frail elderly people vary widely in the level of resources they need to enable them to cope with a given set of problems. If objective tests are used to determine financial entitlements according to predetermined rules (the insured entitlement or 'indemnity' model), and if these tests are devised to ensure that beneficiaries get enough to cover their needs, there will inevitably be a proportion of 'good copers' who will be entitled to receive more benefits than they actually need. Thus the insured entitlement model for funding care for people living in their own homes has an inbuilt tendency towards inefficiency (failure to target resources to needs). That is a price worth paying where transparency of entitlement is seen as a high priority, and insurance companies providing long-term care insurance and similar private funding products have all chosen to offer defined cash entitlements triggered by objective tests, in the form of Activities of Daily Living (ADLs). They have adopted the 'indemnity' model because they judge that few individuals would buy insurance without that assurance of objectivity. As long-term care insurance develops, insurers may be faced with pressure to introduce self-certification for benefits, which may further reinforce inflationary tendencies. Self-certification is advocated by disability organisations and has been introduced by the government as a means of triggering some social security benefits for disabled people.

In contrast, expenditure control assumes a greater importance in the state-funded sector and this is most effectively achieved by a 'rationing by need' model of triggering benefits, in which reimbursement is limited to individually tailored packages of care which emerge out of an informal negotiating process dominated by discretionary judgements made by professionals operating within a budget. The latter model leaves individual entitlements ill defined, but resources are better targeted to needs and the model is less subject to inflationary pressures.

Another inflationary effect of private insurance funding, or indeed any form of third-party funding of long-term care, arises from the more formal methods of paying for care that funding agencies are likely to require. Most private care for people living in their own homes is presently arranged on a cash basis, with little if any payment of overheads, national insurance or tax. Current tax regulations, however, cause more formal billing procedures to be adopted because, in order to avoid tax on benefit payments, long-term care insurers must contract directly with the care provider and may not pay benefits in cash direct to the insured person (see p 134).

STATE FUNDING CONSTRAINTS

The effectiveness of state budgetary controls is the single most important factor which will determine the level of spending on long-term care in the future. The importance of effective budget-capping is crystal clear in the NHS, where the UK has kept costs down to about 6 per cent of GDP compared with figures of 8 or 9 per cent for acute health care elsewhere in Europe and approaching 12 per cent in the USA. In the long-term care sector, the UK has just moved from a mainly open-ended state financing system, through Income Support, to the present budget-capped system of central government grants to local authorities. There can be little doubt that the new system will bring to an end the rapid growth in state funding of long-term care in care home settings experienced over the previous decade. Moreover, starting from a higher baseline than in the past, it should prove possible for the state

to keep long-term care budget increases at or below the level necessary to keep pace with demographic change.

EFFICIENCY
Part of the rationale of the 1993 community care reforms was to promote more efficient use of limited state care resources. The perverse
incentive for state-funded individuals to enter a care home rather than
to seek support services while living in their own homes has been
largely removed (though not entirely – see Chapter 2), and transfer of
budgets to local authorities has created an environment in which case
management techniques of the kind pioneered at the University of
Kent (see p 79) can be widely applied. An evaluation by the Personal
Social Services Research Unit has shown that frail elderly people at
the margin of requiring care in NHS or care home settings can be
cared for cost-effectively in their own homes through the provision of
case-managed packages of intensive day and domiciliary services
(Davies and Challis, 1986). There are undoubtedly opportunities for
reducing costs through case management, but there is a growing
recognition that, above a given level of disability, the delivery of care
in people's own homes dispersed over a wide geographical area
rapidly becomes more expensive than delivering care in settings
where a number of dependent elderly people are concentrated at a
single location.

Because long-term care is, by its nature, a low-tech activity, tech-
nology-led inflation does not assume the importance that it does in the
area of acute health care. On the other hand, the prospects for cost-
reducing technology, through substitution of capital for labour, are
limited. The scope for technological innovation is probably greatest
with care services for people living in their own homes, particularly in
the area of communications where dispersed alarm systems may ultimately grow into much more far-reaching systems for requesting and
delivering care services. Whether such new technology will on balance be cost-reducing or cost-increasing is not yet clear.

In summary, there are some inflationary pressures which will push
long-term care costs upwards. But there are also some countervailing
deflationary pressures, particularly through capping of local authority
budgets. On balance, there is little to support the alarmist scenario of

more rapid than expected inflation pushing long-term care expenditure in the UK substantially above the 'best estimate' projections set out above.

Moreover, in contrast to acute health care, the independent long-term care sector can be characterised as highly competitive. There are no powerful professional vested interests, there are no natural local monopolies like hospitals, and barriers to entry on the supply side are, and are likely to remain, fairly low.

7 Policy issues

The aim of this chapter is to review and assess the policy options open to a government wishing to place the funding of long-term care on an equitable, rational and affordable basis and to forestall any problems that may emerge as a consequence of well-known demographic trends.

It would be vain to attempt to prescribe a single 'best' set of policies on technical grounds, since different approaches to state financing are ultimately political and bound up in differing ideologies. Rather, the aim here is to highlight those options which seem to hold the greatest promise, which may potentially command a wide range of political support, and which may stand up to scrutiny in the national debate which is urgently needed on the financing of long-term care for elderly people in Britain. Some of the policy options identified can be described as radical, some would involve relatively minor 'fine tuning' of existing policies, and some call for the application of fairly novel concepts in the context of existing arrangements.

▬ What would Beveridge have recommended with hindsight?

Earlier chapters have shown how the bulk of state funding for long-term care for elderly people in Britain has always consisted of selective, means-tested provision funded out of taxation. The postwar creation of the welfare state did nothing to alter this. If, however, William Beveridge had been writing his plan for Britain's welfare state in 1993, rather than 1942, how might he have differed in his approach to social insurance for the long-term care of elderly people? Would he, in the light of late twentieth-century demographic projections, have recommended moving long-term care out of the 'sweep up' category of services to be paid for through means-tested benefits? One of Beveridge's basic tenets was that individuals should receive benefits in return for contributions. The central principle of his plan was universal benefits for the eligible population. Selective, means-tested, non-contributory state benefits were to become no more than a safety net for the minority of people inadequately covered by contributory social insurance.

Beveridge's vision of a small, residual role for means-tested benefits has never, however, been realised. Only one in 33 Britons were dependent on means-tested benefits in 1948; in 1990 the figure was one in eight. The initially minor cracks in the edifice of the contributory welfare state, which Beveridge envisaged would be filled by means-tested National Assistance, have become ever-widening fissures as a consequence of fundamental changes in British society. Speaking in the House of Commons debate on the Social Security Bill in November 1992, on the 50th anniversary of the Beveridge report, Malcolm Wicks identified three particular groups which were always poorly covered by contributory benefits, but which have grown from being small minorities in Beveridge's day to substantial sections of society now: working women (particularly those in part-time employment); people whose marriages or partnerships have broken down (particularly single parents); and frail elderly people in need of long-term care services. In the case of long-term care, Wicks declared himself undecided on the various policy options, but argued strongly for a more wide-ranging public debate on what the welfare state should offer:

> If Beveridge were producing his plan today, and the Secretary of State were responding to it, I wonder whether Beveridge might say that one of the insurable risks of modern society should be the need for care in old age. That should be on our agenda . . . (Wicks, 1992)

Options for state financing of long-term care need to be discussed in the context of the evolution of Britain's social security system as a whole. The tendency during recent decades has been to dilute the contributory element of financing and move towards selective rather than universal benefits. Pressure on public sector budgets created by the massive funding deficits that became apparent in 1992 has generated calls for a further shift towards selectivism from right of centre politicians. There have even been recent indications of support on the left of the political spectrum for the idea that a degree of selectivity should be introduced into state pensions, in order to enhance their value for those with no other source of income. Frank Field (1992), for example, writing in a Fabian Society paper, has argued:

> As far as I am concerned there would never be any question of taking the right to that [state retirement] pension away from anyone. But in the scenario I describe [passing control of occupational pension funds to trades unions] it would be legitimate to question whether, each year, the entire pensioner population should have their old age pension upgraded in line with prices.

The erosion of the principle of universalism stems in part from increasing prosperity during the long postwar boom. At the inception of the welfare state in 1948, universal pensions were well targeted because most old people were poor. But this is no longer so, and it weakens the argument for universal benefits for elderly people in general.

If there were to be a new Beveridge report now, one may speculate whether it would recommend revitalisation of the original contributory principle of National Insurance, implying perhaps the creation of a new contributory benefit for long-term care, or whether it would recommend abandonment of the idea of contributory benefits in favour of targeted, means-tested benefits paid from general taxation, implying acceptance of the status quo for long-term care? And what should the role of the government be, if any, in encouraging private financing of long-term care?

The key policy questions on state financing of long-term care for elderly people are as follows:

1   Is long-term care a risk that the state should cover?

2   Is there a case for non-means-tested social insurance for long-term care?

3   Should the government encourage private financial provision for care in old age, and if so, how?

4   Is the balance right between funding of services and income supplementation?

5   How should the government promote efficiency and individual choice in long-term care services?

All these questions concern the structure of the financing system, which is the central concern of this book. The question of the adequacy of public sector budgets for long-term care, under specific financing arrangements, is a topic for a different sort of book and has deliberately been avoided here.

▬ Is long-term care a risk that the state should cover?

The underlying rationale of the welfare state is that the state has a responsibility to promote the welfare of its citizens by protecting them from the financial consequences of certain life risks which may not be readily insurable. For these risks, the state itself takes on the role of insurer or may legislate for compulsory private insurance. To what extent should long-term care be accepted as one of those risks? The state provides a basic safety net for dependent elderly people who are unable to look after themselves, and that entitlement is not at issue. But should the state offer a greater degree of protection for one of the major life risks, needing care in old age?

At present, outside the basic safety net, the state leaves the risk to lie where it falls and the minority of people who require long-term care in a care home must spend down virtually all their assets and income before becoming eligible for state assistance. The issue of whether the state should provide greater financial protection against the risk of needing such care by modifying or abandoning means-testing is considered in the following section on selective versus universal state financing.

Support for carers

Financial protection for people who come to need long-term care is not, however, the only issue, and arguably not even the main one. The massive amount of unpaid care provided by family and friends has already been noted (see *Table 3*). If the time spent on such care were to be valued at £7 per hour the resulting estimate of cost, at £32.5 billion, would dwarf the £9.1 billion spent on formal, paid long-term care services for people aged 65 and over.

As noted on page 49, the burden of care is not spread evenly and can be very severe indeed for a significant minority, particularly long-term, co-resident carers. Apart from Invalid Care Allowance, which is only available for carers who are under the age of 65 when they first claim and whose income does not exceed certain specified limits, the state provides no special assistance or compensation. It has also been noted (pp 46–48) that co-resident carers usually get little local authority support because of 'informal selectivism' which selectively concentrates local authority resources on disabled and elderly people who live alone.

Heavily involved carers are thus severely disadvantaged: they are denied significant protection from the state and have no realistic private insurance alternative. Of all the gaps in the welfare state's arrangements for covering long-term care risks, this appears to merit the most urgent review on grounds of equity. In a report for the Social Security Advisory Committee (Glendinning and McLaughlin, 1993) the authors found that state financial support for unpaid carers is lower in the UK than in other European countries. They recommended a number of policy initiatives that could help to improve the financial situation of unpaid carers in the UK:

- raising the level of Invalid Care Allowance payments for carers towards the levels of care allowances elsewhere in Europe to maintain the income of carers and sustain relationships between carers and the people they care for;

- instituting tax allowances synchronised with cash payments for both carers and people with care needs to help carers to combine care-giving with employment;

- setting up employment protection measures, on the lines of current maternity protection and provision, to encourage caring, enhance public revenues and support equality of opportunity for carers;

- encouraging the increasing numbers of able-bodied older people, who are currently excluded from any financial help in the UK, to provide help to their slightly older counterparts needing care.

On public expenditure grounds, too, there *may* be a case for increased financial support for carers, if such support can be shown to have the effect of preventing them withdrawing from caring, with the catastrophic effect that would have on local authority care budgets. It should be stressed that there is no evidence on the degree to which carers' commitment to caring is influenced by financial considerations – and this is a suitable topic for research – but it is at least plausible that well-targeted government spending on support for carers might lead to lower public spending overall. For example, a non-means-tested 'Severe Dependency Premium', payable with a revamped Invalid Care Allowance, where the cared-for person had been assessed by a local authority as being on the borderline of needing residential or nursing home care, might prove to be a cost-effective addition to the range of state benefits.

In contrast, as is shown below, it is difficult to envisage how the introduction of financial incentives to encourage uptake of private financial products for long-term care funding could achieve any net reduction in public expenditure. On both equity and efficiency grounds, enhanced benefits for carers have a stronger claim than existing private financial products for long-term care for any government finances that may be available.

There is also a strong case for channelling any additional resources for carers through the social security system rather than through local authority care budgets (see below).

▪ Is there a case for non-means-tested social insurance?

For the purposes of this book, the term social insurance is used in its broadest possible sense to cover any financing system for long-term care in which most or all individuals are required by government to pool the risk of long-term care costs, whether through taxation, earmarked National Insurance or even compulsory private insurance, and where the benefits to individuals needing care are not subject to a means test. Another book could be filled with a discussion of variations on the theme of social insurance, but for present purposes the aim is simply to identify the principal consequences of a hypothetical change from the present system of selective, means-tested state funding.

The case for social insurance rather than means-tested state benefits remains essentially the same as it was in the early decades of this century when it was a live issue in the context of a range of social benefits, in particular pensions. The case for non-means-tested pensions was argued and finally won in Britain principally on the grounds that means-testing imposed a penalty on thrift and self-reliance. Thrifty individuals received no state pensions until they had exhausted their resources while the spendthrift, having saved nothing, got immediate financial assistance from the state. Apart from the unfairness, the champions of social insurance emphasised the harmful effects of means-testing in discouraging individuals, friendly societies and progressive employers from putting money aside for retirement. In this sense, the replacement of means-tested with non-means-tested benefits would be, for long-term care now as it was for pensions in the past, a change wholly consistent with Conservative philosophy.

Public expenditure cost

The overriding issue, however, is the public expenditure cost. Whether additional finance for non-means-tested benefits were raised by taxation, earmarked National Insurance or compulsory private insurance premiums would make no difference to the fact that it would represent a significant new compulsory claim on individual income at a time when the government's long-term aim is to increase the proportion of income available for individuals' discretionary use.

How large this claim would be depends on the extent of any move away from selectivity. The radical option of creating a comprehensive new entitlement to benefits to pay the basic cost of long-term care regardless of income or assets would be the most expensive. As noted above, the state currently pays about 70 per cent of Britain's estimated £9.1 billion (1992) spending on long-term care services for elderly people. If the state moved towards universal funding it might ultimately pick up 90 per cent of the cost, implying an additional cost in taxes or compulsory social insurance payments of some £1.8 billion at 1992 prices (0.3 per cent of GDP). With population ageing, the extra cost of comprehensive, universal state funding would rise over time (see *Table 14*). By the peak demand year of 2051 the additional cost would be 0.7 per of GDP. In fact, this probably understates the future *additional* cost of a universal funding scheme to the exchequer because, in the absence of any government initiative, the state-funded element of long-term care can be expected to fall below the current 70 per cent as increasing numbers of property owners are disqualified from receiving state benefits for residential and nursing home care. No allowance is made for this factor in *Table 14*.

Universal state funding for long-term care would undoubtedly, therefore, be an expensive programme. Whether it is affordable is a political decision, which has not yet been informed by any proper national debate. If the outcome of the debate were in favour of universal state funding, then a secondary set of questions would have to be asked about where the money should come from – out of general taxation like the NHS or through the contributory National Insurance fund – and whether provision should be made for opting out into private long-term care insurance schemes.

Table 14 Projected percentage of GDP absorbed by long-term care of elderly people*

	Overall national spending % of GDP	State spending at present (70% of total) % of GDP	State spending if benefits universal (90% of total) % of GDP	Cost of shift from selective to universal benefits % of GDP
1992	1.5	1.0	1.3	0.3
2001	1.7	1.2	1.6	0.4
2051	3.5	2.5	3.2	0.7

* Assumes that age-specific service use will remain constant and that long-term care service prices will rise in line with GDP per capita.

The method of projection is the same as that described on page 39, *Table 3*.

Access to services

Before addressing the question of means-tested versus universal benefits, it is necessary to ask what are the objectives of the welfare state in
financing long-term care. In the broadest terms, the twin objectives are
to ensure access to a reasonable minimum level of service and to distribute taxpayers' money equitably. The first of these objectives, access, is not really at issue in this context because it can be achieved
equally well under a means-tested or a non-means-tested regime. The
minimum access objective is broadly achieved under the present system, in the sense that few if any frail elderly people in extreme need
completely slip through the safety net, and access would not necessarily be enhanced by replacement of this system with a non-means-
tested social insurance model of state financing. Indeed, abandonment
of means-testing may militate against access, in the sense that whatever resources were allocated to the programme would have to be
spread among a larger number of eligible people. Canada, for example, operates a social insurance model for long-term care but its flat-
rate charges are such that many less well-off Canadians do not have
access to single rooms (see pp 83–84). The choice of means-tested versus universal benefits rests, therefore, on considerations of cost and
equity alone.

Inter-generational equity

The first equity-based argument against selective state funding is that
people who find they are ineligible for state benefits may complain
they have been sold a false prospectus by the state. Having paid their
taxes and National Insurance throughout their working lives, or having spouses who did, they may feel understandably aggrieved when
they find that the free NHS long-stay nursing care that they may have
expected is no longer available and that, if they enter a non-NHS care
home, they have to spend down their assets before they qualify for
state help.

There is some validity in this argument. The NHS has certainly reduced its provision of long-stay geriatric beds at a time when the population of very old people has been rising. The counter-argument,

however, is that it has been quite clear from the inception of the welfare state in 1948 that access to the bulk of state provision of long-term care outside people's own homes has been means-tested. Up to the 1970s, local authorities provided most of such means-tested care, and more recently it has been provided by independent care homes. If the current elderly generation of property owners does have a valid complaint, it is that the balance of services has shifted to their disadvantage, not that a whole new funding principle has been introduced. What has happened is that many if not most of the frail elderly people at the upper end of the dependency range, who would have received 'free' NHS long-stay care under the pattern of services 40 years ago, now have to pay for their long-term care in a local authority or independent care home.

More broadly, the issue here is about inter-generational equity. David Thompson (1992) refers to an implicit welfare contract between generations, under which those of working age are willing to be net payers in the expectation of receiving rewards later. Thompson argues, however, that the consistency and reciprocity which should underpin these inter-generational transfers have not been delivered. Changes in taxes, social insurance contributions and benefits result from political imperatives rather than considerations of social justice. One generation may be advantaged at the expense of another. As a consequence there may be a loss of confidence in collective action, increased anxiety about whether future security can be delivered, and indifference to the plight of the poor. Using data largely from New Zealand, Thompson maintains that those born between 1920 and 1945, whom he calls the 'welfare generation', and particularly those born after 1930, have been exceptionally privileged. This generation benefited from high employment and welfare policies designed to support families, and it will continue to benefit in old age in the 1990s and 2000s as a consequence of an inversion of social security priorities from supporting the young to supporting the old. The idea that today's generation of British elderly can similarly be characterised as privileged would be vigorously opposed by many commentators. Hill (1992), for example, found no empirical evidence to support the notion of a welfare generation in Britain. The important point to emerge from Thompson's analysis, however, which does seem to apply equally to Britain, is that it has proved difficult for the state equitably to sustain the implicit welfare contract between generations. Two diametrically opposite conclusions may be drawn from Thompson's analysis. One is that special efforts should be made to revitalise the welfare state by resisting changes in taxes and benefits that run counter to equity between generations. The other is that we should accept that governments will never be able to deliver their side of the implicit welfare contract and that state welfare provision should therefore be replaced as far as possible by private welfare provision through funded insurance schemes, in which beneficiaries have defined property rights which offer a better guarantee of consistency and reciprocity than pay-as-you-go state social insurance schemes.

Intra-generational equity

In addition to the issue of inter-generational equity, there is also the question of equity between different members of the same elderly generation. This may be illustrated by imaginary stereotypes of two frail elderly next-door neighbours, both widows, each of whose husbands formerly had the same sort of job. One has lived a frugal life, accumulating savings to give a little extra income, and buying a small house in the expectation of passing it on to the children. The other has always been a spendthrift; she rents from a housing association, is wholly dependent on state benefits, and expects to die broke. If they both need a home help/home care worker, one will probably have to pay from her savings while the other will get it free. And if they enter the same care home, one will have to sell her house to pay for care but the other will have all her fees paid immediately by the local authority. Probably the majority of people in Britain today would view the situation described as manifestly unfair, and that might be seen as an argument in favour of more universal benefits for long-term care. A substantial minority of the British population would not, however, view the situation described as inequitable at all. Divergent political philosophies probably make any search for consensus on this question fruitless.

Should all 'health' care be excluded from means-testing?

Another argument, for a more limited shift away from means-testing, is that the state ought at least to pay for all *health* care irrespective of means. The definition of health would include all nursing care, which is now more frequently provided on a means-tested basis in independent nursing homes than free in NHS long-stay hospitals. According to this argument there is a contradiction at the heart of current government policy which needs to be resolved. On the one hand the new system of state funding introduced in April 1993 provides for local authorities to pay for nursing care, subject to a means test. At the same time the Secretary of State for Health acknowledges that the NHS has responsibility to pay for nursing care, if the individual concerned insists. The fourth report of the Social Security Committee (HMSO, 1991) reiterates the unequivocal Department of Health acceptance that:

> Health authorities have a responsibility under the National Health Service Act 1977 to provide nursing care for those who cannot or do not wish to pay for it. Department of Health guidance is clear that people should not be discharged into private nursing homes if they have no wish to pay . . .

But the reality, according to the Committee, is that many hospitals have not adhered to the spirit of the Department of Health guidance. In any case, there are not sufficient long-stay places in NHS hospitals to give people the choice. An inequitable situation has therefore developed in which those elderly people who find themselves in NHS hospitals receive their long-term care free while others with the same nursing needs who find themselves in independent nursing homes have to pay according to their means. Equally, it may be argued, it is inequitable and irrational for community health services such as district nursing to be available on a non-means-tested basis while some very similar services provided by local authorities are subject to formal or informal means tests – and for local authority care services for people living in their own homes to be variably means-tested while residential and nursing home care is severely means-tested.

It must be said, however, that the converse argument may be equally valid, that the Department of Health guidance on health authorities' responsibility to provide long-term nursing care may be inappropriate, and that the inequitable treatment of long-stay residents in NHS hospitals and independent nursing homes should be resolved by making long-stay hospital patients pay according to their means.

The underlying issue here is the rationale for some parts of the welfare state, such as medical care and school education, being financed on a universal basis and others, such as housing, being financed on a selective basis. One answer may be that the policy objectives of equality and 'solidarity' are more directly relevant to school education and medical care. The idea, for example, that people should have equal access to the highest quality medical treatment for life-threatening diseases still commands support across a wide spectrum of political opinion. On the other hand, no significant element of the left in Britain has ever proposed that the aim of housing policy should be to attain equality between social classes in the standard of housing. At most, the aim of Labour policy has been to ensure an adequate minimum, for which selective, targeted funding is the appropriate mechanism.

Standing awkwardly in between these extremes is long-term care for elderly people. As it involves elements of both housing and health care, there does not appear to be any overwhelming case in equity either for or against means-tested state financing. Moreover, if Britain is wrong in applying the selective principle to state funding of long-term care, it is an error which is shared with the majority of other OECD countries, some of which apply an even more severe means-testing regime (see Chapter 5).

Distribution of income and wealth

The effect on the distribution of income and wealth needs to be considered. What would be the redistributive effect of replacing means-tested benefits with some form of social insurance for long-term care? One effect would clearly be to redistribute resources in favour of frail elderly people in need of long-term care. But the principal effect, in practice, would be to conserve assets for elderly people to pass on at death. This would be welcomed by those who wish to see wealth, largely in the form of house equity, cascading down generations. But it has to be asked whether it is sensible to cut other public sector spending or raise new taxes to support a programme whose principal effect is to enlarge the pool of often well-off people receiving inheritances on the death of their parents.

Incentives

Finally, what would be the effect on incentives? The view of the political right is that state benefits weaken incentives to work and save in general, though this may be mitigated where there is some visible link between what is contributed and what is taken out in benefits. On this view, a contributory social insurance scheme of the SERPS type for long-term care might be viewed as preferable, or state support for private long-term care insurance (see below). Enhanced state financing may also undermine families' willingness to care for their relatives. In particular, any relaxation of the severity of the assets test for state benefits for residential and nursing home care may reduce the incentive of prospective beneficiaries to keep their elderly parents out of such care. It might, however, ensure that family carers were able to give up caring before their own health was permanently damaged to become another cost for the NHS.

In summary, there are elements of inequity in the existing system of state funding of long-term care, but the case for the state to take on a major new social insurance programme for the financing of long-term care in order to resolve them is by no means clear-cut. If, on balance, it is believed that there is merit in reducing the degree of means-testing for long-term care, the two most practical options open to the state are, first, minor modification of the means-testing regime and, second, introduction of a partial social insurance scheme. These two options are considered next.

Minor modification of the means-testing regime

This option would maintain the means-testing principle, but to modify it in order to relieve its most severe effects. For example, the assets disregard limit of £8,000, beyond which individuals are ineligible for state support to enter residential or nursing home care, might be raised and the tariff income rule might be modified. At present, it is assumed that claimants for state support for residential or nursing home care receive a 'tariff income' of £1 per week for every £250 of capital between £3,000 and £8,000, and this is deducted from any state funding entitlement. Relaxation of these rules would particularly help people with a moderate level of assets who wish to enter a care home where the charges are higher than the local authority is willing to cover, but who are worried that the limited disregard will leave them with insufficient resources over and above state benefits to assure their continued ability to meet the extra charges until death. Another approach may be to limit the application of the means test in those cases where the financial welfare of another individual is adversely affected. For example, if an elderly person jointly owns a property with an individual not covered by the specific capital disregards, that individual may have to dispose of the property in order that the cost of care can be paid. Another example is where an elderly person entering a care home has an occupational pension which has hitherto assured his or her spouse of a good standard of living. But the whole of this occupational pension will be taken into account in determining the charge for care, leaving the spouse with only a basic minimum income. Though there is a clear duty on spouses to support each other, some people may view the operation of the means-testing system in this way as excessively harsh. On the other hand, it should be recognised that this argument amounts to saying that whereas it does not matter if the person in the care home is impoverished as a result of the means test, it *does* matter if the less dependent person's financial position is adversely affected. Other possible measures involving marginal changes to means-testing rules are discussed in the following section on private financial products. Minor modifications like this would go some way towards addressing the intra-generational equity issue, but the other equity issues raised by means-testing would remain unresolved.

Partial social insurance

The most rational policy option, though an expensive one, is the *partial* social insurance model which is used in France and is planned to be adopted in Germany (see p 85). This stands out clearly as a means of resolving many of the equity issues and removing the remaining perverse incentives in the UK state funding system, at a cost which would be less than that of a fully comprehensive social insurance scheme.

A partial social insurance scheme would make long-term care itself a non-means-tested state benefit, subject only to assessment of need, but would continue the present severe means-testing regime for the hotel element of residential and nursing home care. Means-testing of the hotel element would also be extended to NHS long-stay hospitals. At its most rational, the non-means-tested care entitlement would extend to 'social' as well as 'nursing' care in order to avoid the arbitrary distinctions that are currently made between the two, in the UK and elsewhere. In this way, the option of partial social insurance described here is more generous than the system which presently operates in France, where a distinction is made, both for care outside people's own homes and for care for people living in their own homes, between non-means-tested nursing care and means-tested social care.

The merits of such a partial social insurance system would be:

- It would resolve the inter-generational equity issue (where elderly people may feel they are being denied care services that they have paid for in their working lives) by creating an easily understood entitlement to all care services, with no arbitrary distinctions between 'health' and 'social' care.

- It would go some way towards resolving the intra-generational equity issue (where people who have saved for their old age are currently no better off than those who have not).

- It would largely remove the remaining inbuilt perverse incentives within the state funding system, which are caused by means-testing. Local authorities would no longer have a financial incentive to direct owner-occupiers to residential or nursing home care, where they can recover the full cost of care from liquidation of home equity, rather than care services for people living in their own homes, where they cannot. Also, the incentive for families to seek 'free' NHS care in order to save their inheritances would be reduced.

- The community care reforms have already separated out 'care' funding (by local authorities) from 'hotel' services funding (from the Department of Social Security).

The overriding issue, of course, remains the public expenditure cost. Hotel charges for NHS long-stay hospital beds would reduce this cost. This would have the added virtue of creating a more rational system, since it would entirely remove the existing financial incentive for better-off elderly people and their relatives to seek long-term care in an NHS setting rather than elsewhere. There would, of course, be strong political objections to introducing charges for hospital beds as an isolated measure, but presented as part of a package of reforms offering extended social insurance cover for long-term care, objections would carry much less weight.

A likely effect of replacing means-tested with non-means-tested state benefits for long-term care would be to increase the incentives for both the less well-off and the better-off segments of the population to spend on private funding products, though for different reasons. The less well-off segment would be encouraged to spend because their perceived marginal return would cease to be zero, as their state entitlement ceased to be reduced pound for pound by any private benefit income. The better-off segment of the population would probably be encouraged to spend because private funding products would become more affordable. Private products could be designed to top up non-means-tested state entitlements. Only if the government pursued a policy of making state long-term care so good that no one would want to go private would the incentive to buy private funding products sink to zero for the less well-off segment of the population and, in the unlikely event that non-means-tested benefits were set very high, for the better-off segment of the population as well.

The adoption of partial social insurance would also open the way to contracting out arrangements similar to the SERPS opt-out, whereby individuals who wished to opt for an approved private scheme would be able to claim a National Insurance or tax rebate designed to be budget-neutral.

▪ Should the government encourage private funding mechanisms?

The first question is whether private funding mechanisms should be encouraged at all. There is no a priori case for government intervention in the market-place. A clear justification is required in terms of valid public policy objectives. Vague assertions that the state will be unable to fund the rising costs of long-term care in the future are insufficient.

The arguments given in this section are all set in the context of the existing system of means-tested state benefits for residential and nursing home care. If, as a consequence of public debate, the government were to adopt the principle of social insurance for long-term care, then a whole set of other considerations might come into play, including the possibility of tax relief, National Insurance credits or even vouchers to enable people to contract out of any state social insurance scheme that might be introduced into a private sector alternative (as the government has encouraged contracting out of SERPS into private pension schemes). But these considerations simply do not apply under the present means-tested financing system. There is little or no validity in the concept of contracting out of a means-tested system because, following the SERPS analogy, contracting out depends on the state being able to give to people wanting to buy into a private scheme a rebate about equal to the savings accruing to the state scheme as a consequence of opt-out. But since the cost of a means-tested scheme is concentrated among people with few resources (who are unlikely to want to contract out), the savings in state benefits that the state can afford to pass on to better-off people wishing to contract out will be too small to create any significant incentive to do so.

Tax concessions

One policy option that has been canvassed in the context of the present system of means-tested state benefits is to encourage private arrangements to fund long-term care through tax concessions. This might be done by giving income tax relief for long-term care insurance premiums. It might also be done by widening the benefits that can be obtained under current tax concessions for pensions. Tax concessions have often proved to be an effective means of encouraging the rapid growth of new financial products, for example private pensions.

An advantage of tax concessions is that they act as a focus for promoting awareness of issues. The disadvantage is that once concessions have been granted it is difficult to remove them. The other objection in principle is that tax concessions distort the market and can therefore be expected to lead to sub-optimal allocative efficiency.

There are three issues to consider:

- any macro-economic effects of tax concessions;

- whether loss of tax revenue would be justified by reductions in government expenditure on other accounts;

- whether provision for long-term care is something that should be positively encouraged over other forms of consumption.

MACRO-ECONOMIC EFFECTS

Any macro-economic effects of tax concessions are likely to be fairly small. Whether encouraged by tax concessions or not, long-term care funding products will probably develop as a niche market, and any additional flows of savings and expenditure they generate are unlikely to have any significant effect on the overall level of savings or consumption in the economy. Some long-term care funding mechanisms such as long-term care insurance are prefunded plans whose effect would initially be to increase the level of savings in the economy. Others, for example equity release, would not have this effect but might save on Income Support payments. Equity release products might have the most significant macro-economic impact. To the extent that equity release is used to pay for a substantial increase in care services for people living in their own homes, the consumption of the value of housing equity may substantially reduce the projected flow of inherited wealth to younger generations as older generations increase their rates of owner occupation. However, taking all factors into account, there does not appear to be any strong macro-economic case either for or against tax concessions for long-term care funding products.

NET PUBLIC EXPENDITURE SAVINGS FROM TAX CONCESSIONS?
It is not possible to make a convincing case for tax concessions in terms of public expenditure savings, except possibly where the products eligible for tax concessions are specifically targeted on particular segments of society and particular long-term care services. It is sometimes loosely argued that the exchequer must benefit from tax concessions because public money will not have to be spent on individuals who have made their own provision, if and when long-term care is needed. But this fails to take into account the 'dead money' issue. The problem is that tax concessions go not only to those who, as a direct consequence, reduce their consumption of state benefits; they also go to those who would have bought the product anyway, without tax concessions, and to those whose consumption of state benefits is not changed by buying the product. There will be no overall benefit to the exchequer unless the net savings from the former group are greater than the dead money spent on tax concessions to the latter group. Any pay-back to the state is likely to be particularly low in the case of tax concessions for products to fund residential or nursing home care since the people likely to buy such products tend to be those who would not have received means-tested benefits anyway. And even in the case of less severely means-tested services for people living in their own homes, the payoff is unlikely to be sufficient to cover the tax subsidy, unless receipt of tax relief were made conditional on the recipient losing entitlement to state-funded services. But that would be a major step further than simple tax relief. In fact, it is rare for tax concessions to generate overall savings to the exchequer. Long-term care funding products are most unlikely to prove to be an exception to the rule that tax incentives do not give a payoff in terms of reduced government spending.

For example, it is widely recognised within the private medical insurance sector that tax relief on medical insurance premiums for people aged 60 and over simply caused subscribers to switch to eligible policies. The net addition of new subscribers was very small. Although it is not possible to measure the consequent reduction in consumption of NHS services, it was certainly much less than the estimated £40 million of lost tax revenue.

The public expenditure savings case, if any, for tax concessions differs according to the type of long-term care funding product. In the case of long-term care insurance, purchasers cannot at present offset their premiums against income tax. If they could, would the exchequer save money as a result? The answer is almost certainly no, because the great bulk of the tax revenue forgone by the exchequer would probably be dead money. Long-term care insurance would be bought mainly by people in the A, B, C1 groups who are relatively well-off, who typically own their own homes and/or have significant other assets, and would thus be unlikely to qualify for means-tested state funding for residential or nursing home care. It is true that there would be some savings to the exchequer from those people ineligible for means-tested benefits on admission to a care home who spend down their resources and would, in the absence of long-term care insurance benefits, become reliant on state means-tested benefits. Finally, the state would benefit from some increase in inheritance tax on death, since recipients of private long-term care insurance benefits would be less likely to spend down their assets. However, inheritance tax is not a substantial generator of revenue for the state and it has been described as a 'voluntary tax' because there are well-established mechanisms for avoiding liability. In summary, under any reasonable assumptions, the aggregate savings to the exchequer resulting from tax concessions for long-term care insurance would be substantially less than the tax revenue forgone.

Wittenberg (1989), in a Government Economic Service Working Paper, also concluded that the availability of long-term care insurance is unlikely to lead to significant reductions in government expenditure on long-term care outside people's own homes. It is not known what difference tax relief on premiums would make to the uptake of long-term care insurance as this depends on the price elasticity of demand, but Wittenberg concluded that price elasticity would have to be very high indeed for penetration of lower-income bands to rise sufficiently for the reduction in state spending to offset the 'dead money' represented by tax relief for those individuals who would not be eligible for state funding and those who would have bought insurance without tax relief. Moreover, because the time between purchase and receipt of benefits is so long, the state would have to bear the loss of tax revenue for ten or more years before any significant savings on means-tested state benefits fed through.

In the United States, which has a similar system of means-tested public sector benefits for long-term care, Weiner (1992b) comes to a similar conclusion, even where there is a degree of targeting of the tax concession on those most likely to use publicly funded care. Using the Brookings-ICF Long-Term Care Financing Model, and assuming a 20 per cent tax credit on long-term care premiums to be limited to people on relatively moderate incomes, the model projects the cost in forgone tax revenue at $6.4 billion at 1992 prices by the period 2016–2020. Corresponding savings in public spending on means-tested benefits (through Medicaid) are projected at $1.6 billion, so forgone tax revenue would be four times as much as Medicaid savings.

It is possible that the net cost to the state in Britain could be reduced by targeting tax concessions on long-term care insurance products even more precisely on those people who are likely to make use of state-funded long-term care services in the future (low to average income, non-home owners with limited savings). However, apart from the fairness of any such targeting, and the problems of administration, products aimed specifically at less well-off people would not be perceived as a major revenue generator by the financial services sector.

It is difficult, therefore, to conceive of a tax concession for long-term care insurance that would both save the exchequer money and be attractive to the financial services sector.

The same conclusion broadly applies to further tax concessions to encourage pension-linked long-term care funding schemes, though the ratio of tax revenue forgone to means-tested state benefits saved would in this case probably be less disadvantageous to the exchequer: occupational pensions have a broader socio-economic base than potential long-term care insurance subscribers, and more occupational pension holders would be potential users of state means-tested benefits, so the proportion of 'dead money' in the forgone tax revenue would be lower.

The specific tax concessions that have been suggested for pension-linked long-term care products and associated pension annuities are:

- allowing a long-term care pension to be a legitimate benefit entitlement;

- increasing the contribution limit on tax-free earnings that can be placed in a tax-free investment fund, in order to provide more scope for spending on long-term care at maturity;

- extending the benefits from the pension fund which are not taxable in the hands of the pensioner to include any payments for long-term care;

- allowing any annuity purchased to pay for long-term care to benefit from tax-free roll-up of the underlying fund and tax-free payment to the annuitant.

All these suggested concessions combined would make pension-linked long-term care products extremely advantageous from a tax point of view. There may be valid public policy arguments in favour of such advantageous treatment but, for similar reasons to those set out above for long-term care insurance, the prospect of net savings to the exchequer is almost certainly not one of them.

Equity release plans targeted at owner-occupiers on low to average incomes may be the exception to the rule that tax concessions will not deliver net savings to the exchequer. To the extent that equity release purchasers use local authority care services for people living in their own homes, and to the extent that they would use income from equity release to substitute private for state-funded local authority services, tax relief on mortgage interest might give rise to a net saving in public expenditure. Also, low-income purchasers of equity release plans take themselves out of the Income Support bracket, saving state expenditure on that account. At present, mortgage interest tax relief on home income plans for elderly people is limited to £30,000 of borrowing, in common with relief available to other mortgage holders. Age Concern has campaigned for the limit to be increased to £60,000 for home income plans for elderly people. Another brake on this market is that interest has to be paid each year in order to obtain tax relief. Allowing interest on mortgage annuity loans to be rolled up until the annuitant's death and then to be paid from the estate with full tax relief would greatly enhance the appeal of this product.

ARE THERE ANY SPECIAL REASONS FOR ENCOURAGING LONG-TERM CARE SPENDING?

Finally, are there any special reasons why provision for long-term care should be encouraged rather than other forms of consumption? Public subsidies may be justified where the product or service concerned is a public good or where there are 'external' benefits which are not taken into account by individual consumers. An example of an external benefit is the benefit that all members of society derive when individuals seek immunisation against infectious diseases. Again, it would be difficult to make a case for tax concessions on these grounds. It may be that taxpayers would wish to pay for higher spending on long-term care in the context of a social insurance scheme offering equitable benefits to all. The question posed here, however, is whether there is a case for tax concessions to encourage higher spending on long-term care per se. A positive answer to this question would rightly be seen as special pleading.

In summary, therefore, the case for tax concessions to encourage private funding vehicles for long-term care is weak, except possibly for certain highly targeted products. Moreover, most insurance companies involved in developing and marketing long-term care products would broadly accept that, subject to certain modifications, the present tax environment does not unduly hinder the development of financial products for funding long-term care.

Resolving tax anomalies

There is, however, a strong case for measures to resolve existing anomalies in the tax and regulatory treatment of long-term care funding products and for changes in the tax rules which discriminate against certain forms of care.

To summarise the tax anomalies, the embryonic British private long-term care funding market consists of prefunded plans such as long-term care insurance and immediate care plans such as annuities, pseudo-annuities and equity release products. The tax position varies according to the product type. In the case of long-term care insurance, premiums are paid out of taxed income, and if the benefits are paid to the policyholder they too are taxed. But the benefits are not taxable if they are paid direct to the care provider. This is the first anomaly. It may be argued that this particular anomaly has advantages because it encourages a managed approach to third-party care funding, in which the insurer takes responsibility for contracting with the care provider and takes the burden of management of care packages away from the elderly individual. Some elderly people may welcome this. But equally others may wish to have the benefits in their own hands. Moreover, direct payment to care providers is likely to discourage economical forms of home care currently paid for in cash.

Annuities and pseudo-annuities are also paid out of taxed income, but in the absence of any definitive clarification from the Inland Revenue it must be assumed that annuity income spent on care services cannot escape tax, even if paid direct to care providers. In other words – and this is the second anomaly – prefunded plans such as long-term care insurance can escape taxation on benefits while immediate care plans such as annuities cannot.

The third anomaly relates to pension-linked products. It has been noted that when Cannon Lincoln's Oasis Plus plan was introduced in 1991, the Inland Revenue was willing to approve 'low-start, high-finish' personal pension annuities. But the same flexibility was not available for the much larger number of people who have occupational pensions. Since the withdrawal of Inland Revenue approval of the Oasis Plus plan, representatives of the financial services sector have argued that this decision should be reversed. They have also argued that the original anomaly should be ended and that it should be possible in principle for all people with pension rights, not just those with personal pensions, to benefit from tax-free payments into the pension fund and tax-free accumulation of the investment fund, and to select an income where the benefits increase in very old age or on prior severe disability.

Three specific recommendations on the tax and regulatory position can be made here.

BENEFITS PAID TO POLICYHOLDERS OR CARE PROVIDERS

All except one of the long-term care insurance plans which have been launched on the market since 1991 have provided for benefits to be paid direct to the care provider under contract with the insurance company. The reason stressed in product literature is to take the burden of administration away from the elderly person in need of care services. This is a valid argument, and payment direct to care providers will also facilitate the development of managed care procedures which may enhance value for money. But the real reason for payment being made direct to care providers is that, if paid to the policyholder, the benefits would be taxable as income – in the same way as benefits paid under income replacement schemes such as permanent health insurance. Thus tax rules which were originally devised to meet other situations are driving product development in long-term care insurance. It may be being driven in an appropriate direction for the majority of policyholders, but not necessarily for all. It would enhance choice if long-term care insurance benefits paid to subscribers were exempt from income tax in the same way as benefits paid to care providers. It would also be anti-inflationary, by encouraging the continued use of cash payments by recipients of benefits themselves to access low-cost services.

PERSONAL PENSIONS AND OCCUPATIONAL PENSIONS

Until a recent reversal of rules by the Inland Revenue, people who had personal pensions had greater flexibility to use their pension rights to fund long-term care than those who had occupational pensions. It had been agreed, under the Cannon Lincoln plan, that when a personal pension matured the individual could opt to forgo some of the initial value of the annuity that he or she bought with the accumulated fund in return for an enhancement in the event of needing long-term care. Negotiations had also started with the Inland Revenue to extend this principle to allow the use of any appropriate formula for calculating the annuity enhancement allowable, including an amount equivalent to the actual cost of care. It was also argued by financial services interests that people with occupational pensions should enjoy the same flexibility. Existing regulations limit occupational pensions to two-thirds of final salary and this cannot be varied at different times in the life of the pension. A case was put to the Inland Revenue that as long as the actuarial value of the pension is the same then the timing of payments should not matter. In other words, if a pool of individual risks are considered together and the payments over the life of the occupational pensions do not *on average* exceed two-thirds of final salary, it should be possible for the limit to be breached for defined purposes – such as funding long-term care. In the event, however, the Inland Revenue resolved the personal–occupational pension anomaly by disallowing low-start, high-finish pensions for both personal and occupational pensioners.

There is a strong case for this decision to be reversed and for regulations to be amended to allow people with either personal or occupational pensions to have the flexibility to fund long-term care by varying their revenue flows over time. More generally, there is a case for establishing the principle that all people with pension entitlements should, on retirement, be able to select the form in which they receive their pension benefits from a menu of approved options.

ROLLED-UP MORTGAGE INTEREST

There is a case for allowing interest on mortgage annuity loans to be rolled up until the annuitant's death and then paid from the estate with full tax relief. At present, interest has to be paid each year in order to obtain tax relief. A minor change in the rules would encourage people living in their own homes who need expensive care services to use the equity in their owner-occupied homes to pay for them.

Each of these recommendations is presently being pursued by organisations within the financial services sector, acting individually or in concert. Inland Revenue officers and Treasury officials will probably be the key participants in determining whether or not the anomalies in the tax treatment of long-term care funding products are resolved. There are areas, however, where a debate at the political level is required. In particular, there would have to be political will in order to introduce any tax concessions, improvements in tax flexibility or special modifications to the normal means-testing rules that might be proposed to encourage financial products targeted at specific client groups making use of particular long-term care services.

Financial products which complement state entitlements

Because of the high cost of comprehensive private long-term care funding products, an alternative approach to product development by the financial services sector may be to devise relatively low-cost plans which would aim to top up state funding entitlements. Such plans might provide, for example, for extra privately purchased domiciliary services for someone already in receipt of local authority domiciliary services. Or they might provide for an additional sum of money for individuals receiving state-funded residential or nursing home care, to enable them to have a wider choice of home. Such top-up products would not work under present state funding arrangements because, in the case of care home residents, any benefit from a private funding plan would reduce the amount of local authority and/or Income Support funding pound for pound. The only way of avoiding this at present is for the top-up product to be arranged by the family, in which case the benefits will not be counted in the means test. In the case of care services for people living in their own homes, too, receipt of private benefits may reduce people's allocation of local authority resources – and indeed access to other state benefits such as free sight tests. What would be required, therefore, would be a modification of current means-testing principles such that private long-term care plan benefits would be disregarded in determining eligibility for state funded benefits.

In the United States, where many complementary private/public funding initiatives are being debated and tested at state level, the best known example is the Connecticut Health Care Partnership. Under the Connecticut scheme, an individual who has taken out an approved private long-term care plan would claim for care in a care home under that plan for as long as entitlement lasts – say one or two years. If the individual were still alive at the end of that period, he or she would claim Medicaid in the ordinary way. The difference at this stage is that, under the Connecticut plan, for every dollar that has already been spent under the approved private plan, Medicaid would disregard a dollar of assets in the means test. For example, an individual who had received $50,000 in private long-term care benefits would have the first $50,000 of assets disregarded in a subsequent claim for Medicaid benefits. These assets could then either be conserved, to be passed on to heirs, or used to top up the basic Medicaid contribution to fees.

The advantages claimed for the Connecticut partnership are:

- It leads to more affordable, one-year and two-year long-term care policies and thus greatly reduces the financial barriers to making private provision.

- It allows stringent regulations to be attached to qualifying policies, in the interests of consumer protection.

- It allows people to conserve assets and thus avoid impoverishment by long-term care expenses.

- Limited entitlements to have assets disregarded in the means test work out less costly in tax revenue terms than complete abandonment of means-testing, as in a social insurance programme.

A whole variety of similar products might be developed in the UK context, similar in the sense that they give people partial exemption from the normal means test, whether for residential or nursing home care or care for people living in their own homes. A prerequisite would be discussions between the government, the financial services sector and consumer groups with a view to creating a clear framework of rules under which such complementary products might qualify for means-testing concessions.

One hypothetical financial product, for example, is a single premium delayed annuity, which would pay the full cost of residential or nursing home care after (say) two years but would allow the individual to claim state support in the interim. It would probably fall foul of divestment rules on capital at present. The hypothetical product would enable an asset-rich, income-poor entrant to a care home to spend the bulk of his or her assets on buying the annuity, to qualify for state funding until the annuity starts, and to use the £3,000 of disregarded assets and any family contribution to pay for a more expensive care home than the local authority would normally cover. A deferred annuity such as this would place the private funding at the back end of the scheme rather than the front end as in the Connecticut partnership, but otherwise the effect would be similar. It would make (partial) private provision more affordable at a cost to public funds which is higher than under the present means-testing arrangements but lower than under a social insurance scheme which abandoned means-testing altogether.

There are, however, equity objections to all such initiatives designed specifically to stimulate the private financial services sector. Why, it may be asked, should individuals who happen to have purchased approved long-term care financing products be exempted from ordinary means tests while others are not? More broadly – and this objection applies equally to the complete abandonment of means tests – is conservation of assets for beneficiaries an appropriate aim of public policy? There are also efficiency objections. Linking means test exemptions to approved financial products might be viewed as an artificial stimulus to the financial services sector, the marketing and administrative costs of which must be borne by subscribers.

Compulsory private long-term care insurance

Compulsory private long-term care insurance would only become an option if a decision in principle had been taken to move away from a means-tested state funding system to a non-means-tested system based on the insurance principle. Having taken that decision in principle, the coalition partners in the German government recently debated the merits of putting it into effect through the social insurance structure or through compulsory private insurance. In the event, the former was chosen.

In principle, there need be little difference between social insurance and compulsory private insurance. Both involve an additional mandatory claim on personal resources where none existed before. People on low incomes might be brought into a compulsory private insurance scheme through state-funded 'top-ups' of premiums. Both social insurance and compulsory private insurance could be run on the same rules and with similar benefit triggers. In practice, however, a compulsory private insurance scheme, or a contracted-out alternative to otherwise mandatory social insurance, would probably use objective criteria such as ADLs to trigger benefits. This would have the merit of transparency, but the disadvantage of being inflation-prone, as indicated on pages 78–79. In contrast, a social insurance scheme in Britain would probably use a 'rationing by need' model of triggering benefits, in which individually tailored packages of care emerge out of an informal negotiating process dominated by the discretionary judgements of professionals operating within a budget. The latter model leaves individual entitlements ill defined, but is less subject to inflationary pressures.

Summary

A public debate is urgently needed to weigh the balance of advantages and disadvantages of means-tested and non-means-tested systems of long-term care funding. The debate would also serve to clarify in the public mind the distinction between non-means-tested NHS services and means-tested long-term care services and make people with significant resources of their own fully aware of how little they can expect in terms of state support for long-term care. At the very least this would help people to take rational decisions about what provision, if any, to make for themselves.

Any debate is likely to conclude that there is no case for tax concessions to encourage private financial products for long-term care, though there *is* a strong case for ending a number of anomalies in the tax treatment of different financial products. There are equity objections to stimulating private financial products designed to complement state funding through the creation of exceptions to normal means-testing rules, though the relatively limited cost of such exceptions may be justified if they are targeted on individuals who are particularly disadvantaged by the present means-testing regime.

The scope for the private sector to take over the burden of long-term care funding from the public sector is limited. The evidence from the UK and other countries is that prefunded private financial products which offer comprehensive long-term care cover are too expensive to envisage voluntary purchase replacing a substantial proportion of state funding in the foreseeable future. And while state financing for long-term care remains means-tested, there is no validity in the concept of encouraging contracting out into a private sector scheme. The main justification for encouraging private sector initiatives, for example by resolving the tax anomalies, is that they increase choice and may improve the quality of life and peace of mind of the minority who can afford them.

▬ Balance between funding of services and income supplementation

As noted in Chapter 3, there are two parallel streams of state funding for long-term care in the UK today. The larger of the two streams is channelled through third parties (specifically local and health authorities) to pay for defined services used by their clients. The smaller stream is channelled through social security payments such as Income Support, Attendance Allowance, Disability Living Allowance and, until recently, Independent Living Fund payments per elderly people. These are all paid direct to individuals who may spend the benefit at their discretion, whether on care services or on goods and services apparently unrelated to care.

Given the wide variation in individuals' abilities to cope with given degrees of disability, third-party funding agencies which ration resources within fixed budgets are in a much better position to match resources to individual needs. The process of resource allocation, however, inevitably lacks transparency. Social security benefits, in contrast, use objective tests to determine financial entitlements according to predetermined rules. Transparency is high but such benefits are relatively poor at targeting needs. It is for this reason that Sir Roy Griffiths (HMSO, 1988a) summarily dismissed the option of extending social security benefits to pay for community care:

> Our social security system is designed to provide a standard range of benefits for large numbers of people against objective tests of entitlement. It is not an appropriate system for the direct provision of individually tailored packages of support within a finite community care programme.

The option did, however, get support from the Wagner Committee (HMSO, 1986):

We have been much attracted by the idea of issuing Community Care Allowances to people with special needs, to be used by them to procure care services of their choice. The allowance could be used either to recruit help in the home, or to enter a residential home or – if preferred – could be banked with the area social services office where a nominated social worker could assemble a package of care services.

The social security funding principle is most appropriate where large numbers of individuals receive fairly small sums, where the objective of the benefit is as much compensation as service provision, and where the range of relevant service provision may be too wide to define easily. On these grounds, social security entitlements seem to be the preferred means of channelling money to carers.

There is also an equity reason for channelling any additional state financial support for carers through the social security system rather than local authorities. This can best be illustrated by reference to the acute health care sector, where there is a more extensive literature on the implications of rationing and prioritisation under a fixed budget. In Britain, health economists have argued that maximisation of QALYs (Quality Adjusted Life Years) subject to budget constraints is the appropriate criterion for rationing limited health care resources. This may seem unobjectionable, but ultimately what it means is that people with certain illnesses, where the cost in relation to expected benefits is very high, may receive nothing at all. In the United States, a health care rationing method proposed in the State of Oregon provides for precisely that, by excluding from reimbursement any intervention with an expected benefit to cost ratio below a given point. In essence, this amounts to saying that some people, who happen to have conditions whose treatments rank low, should have no entitlement to health care. Though this may be consistent with maximisation of utility across society as a whole, it raises serious questions about the rights of individuals.

In the case of long-term care, prioritisation by local authority social services departments appears to be concentrating limited resources on the most highly dependent elderly people. Those whose care requirements are low may receive little if any local authority care resources and, where there are co-resident carers, this tendency is reinforced by the 'informal selectivism' adopted by local authorities which selectively denies statutory services to clients with a carer.

There is a case, therefore, for carers – and particularly co-resident, long-term carers who are among those most disadvantaged by the existing arrangements for funding long-term care – to receive any additional help through the social security system, where defined rules of entitlement prevent the inequitable prioritisation that may take place within third-party state funding agencies such as local authorities.

■ Promotion of individual choice in long-term care

Concern about individual choice in long-term care relates primarily to the state-funded sector. In the case of residential and nursing home care there were fears that the new system of state financing introduced in April 1993 would give excessive discretionary powers to local authority managers. These fears have been allayed by the government decision to enshrine state-funded individuals' right to choice of care home in statutory guidance. There is no such guidance, however, for services for people living in their own homes, where local authorities continue to exercise purchasing discretion on behalf of their clients. Health authorities also continue to exercise discretion over who gets access and will continue to act as monopoly suppliers of community health services such as district nursing. In this context, the exercise of consumer choice will be heavily dependent on the willingness and ability of street-level rationers of services to take account of consumers' preferences.

The Social Services Committee, in its sixth report (HMSO, 1990c), expressed concern about consumer choice, quoting evidence from Age Concern: 'the element of "choice" for the user will be related not to market forces but to arrangements made by health and local authorities which may have little to do with individuals' perceptions of their own needs' and from David Plank, Director of Social Services in Hounslow: 'at present too much power rests in the hands of the bureaucrats from SSDs and other agencies. The balance of power needs to be adjusted towards disabled people.'

In an Institute of Economic Affairs paper (Laing, 1991) the present author argued for a radical approach to empowering elderly people who use state-funded care services. Local authorities, it was proposed, should continue as the lead agencies for state funding of long-term care and should make funding available only following an assessment of need, as under the current arrangements. But instead of contracting direct with service providers, local authorities should make cash available to service users themselves, to spend on care services of their own choice with the aid, if they wish, of care service 'brokers'. Brokers should be accountable to service users, not to local authorities. An example of such a brokerage scheme, operated by Choice in North London, is described by Kestenbaum (1993a). Those users who do not want to exercise control in any way should be free to leave their cash allocation with the social services department to spend on their behalf.

The proposal draws on the experience of Canadian experiments which show that elderly and disabled people *are* capable of exercising choice effectively in the market-place. Similar conclusions have been drawn from the operation of the Independent Living Fund in Britain. Kestenbaum's (1993a) findings challenge the assumption that disabled people are incapable of exercising effective control and choice over their own care arrangements. Her work also shows that the ability to exercise choice is not confined to younger disabled people but applies to older people as well. Perhaps the most persuasive recent evidence that financial empowerment of disabled people achieves better outcomes comes from Morris (1993). Interviews with 50 people in England found much higher levels of satisfaction among those who could purchase their own care. In contrast, interviewees reported that statutory services were inflexible and failed to enable recipients to go outside their own home or to play a full role in personal relationships. Moreover, the Canadian experiments have shown that such a financing system can achieve the difficult goal of combining economy with choice. A new type of professional, the 'care broker', would be needed, but would often be drawn from the ranks of local authority social services managers, many of whose functions would become redundant.

It is worth pointing out why this model of financial empowerment of the individual is a practical, non-inflationary option for long-term care but is probably unworkable for acute health care (at least for expensive secondary and tertiary health care). The difference lies in the nature of the relationship between service user and provider and the degree of knowledge that consumers can reasonably be expected to have. Typically, consumers of secondary and tertiary health care need these services only occasionally, often urgently, and because of the complexity of medicine they are usually heavily if not wholly dependent on professional advice as to what is the best treatment and who is best able to provide it. In these circumstances it is not really a practicable option to offer cash to individuals who have been assessed as needing treatment, for example, for leukaemia and expect them to balance the cost and quality considerations before buying the service of their choice. In contrast, users of long-term care services are typically regular service users. Provided they are mentally competent, they should have a clear understanding of the services they need in order to maximise their quality of life, provided they have proper, full needs-based assessment, regularly received. Many would argue that they understand their service needs much better than the professionals. Moreover, the balance of power in the relationship between user and care provider is much less one-sided than it often is between doctor and patient. For all these reasons, direct financial empowerment of service users is a practical option for long-term care, though it is not for acute health care.

■ A social market for long-term care

The financial empowerment of elderly care service users would be fully consistent with the 'partial social insurance' system of state funding, identified above as the most promising policy option for resolving inequities and removing the remaining perverse incentives from the present system of state financing. Under such a system, elderly people who are assessed as needing long-term care services would be enabled, if they wished, to receive their entitlement in cash to pay for long-term care services of their own choice. Residents of local authority residential homes would also be eligible for Residential Allowance, paid as part of Income Support to people who qualify on income grounds. This would allow individuals to choose a publicly provided rather than a privately provided care home on the same financial footing. Providers, for their part, would charge for *all* long-term care services at full economic cost, including NHS long-stay beds and both NHS and local authority long-term care services for people in their own homes.

Such a system would create a level playing field for consumers, in which everyone is entitled through partial social insurance to buy the long-term care services of their choice, whether received at home, in care homes or in hospital, and where the hotel element of cost is means-tested in both care homes and NHS hospitals. In essence, what is being suggested here is a fully-fledged social market in long-term care services. Social market advocates argue that the market option of 'exit' (meaning consumers' power to stop buying from a particular provider) is generally superior to 'voice' (meaning the ability to press demands through democratic institutions) as a mechanism for optimising the welfare of individuals. In the case of long-term care there is some convincing evidence to support that view. The market, however, is not only about welfare optimisation in a static world. Economic liberals also emphasise the way markets function as a discovery procedure in a world where tastes and techniques are changing and information is scarce and expensive. Market signals provide an incentive for entrepreneurs to meet unsatisfied needs by creating new possibilities which people did not know existed before (Brittan, 1990). If this view of the market is valid, then financial empowerment of individuals linked with full cost charging by providers should stimulate innovation and create new services to complement and replace the frequently inflexible statutory services currently available for dependent elderly people.

REFERENCES

ABPI (1991) *Agenda for Health: The challenges of ageing.* Association of the British Pharmaceutical Industry, London.

Barry C (1992) Personal communication. Gerontology Data Service, Age Concern Institute of Gerontology.

Berthoud R (1988) 'Using Benefits to Pay for Care at Home', in *Social Security and Community Care,* ed Sally Baldwin, Gillian Parker and Robert Walker. Gower Publishing, Aldershot.

Bone M et al (1992) *Retirement and Retirement Plans.* OPCS, HMSO.

Bosanquet N, Propper C, Laing W (1990) *Elderly Consumers in Europe.* Laing & Buisson, London.

Boyd P (1993) *Social Security Benefits: The new scheme.* Presentation at the 6th Annual Elderly Care Conference organised by Laing & Buisson, March 1993. Laing & Buisson, London.

Bradshaw J, Gibbs I (1988) *Public Support for Private Residential Care.* Gower Publishing, Avebury.

Brittan, S (1990) *A Restatement of Economic Liberation Social Market Foundation.* London.

Buchanan et al (1991) 'Medicaid Payment Policies for Nursing Home Care: A national survey', *Health Care Financing Review,* 13/1.

Daatland S (1990) 'What Are Families For?' *Ageing and Society,* 10/1.

Davies B, Challis D (1986) *Matching Resources to Needs in Community Care.* Gower Publishing, Aldershot.

Davies B, Goddard M (1987) *The Brokerage Only BRITSMO: The BRITSMO concept.* Personal Social Services Unit, University of Kent, Discussion Paper 554.

Department of Employment (1992) 'Civilian Labour Force Composition and Trends', *Employment Gazette*, April 1992.

Department of Health (1992) *Charging for Residential Accommodation Guide.*

DHSS (1987) *Public Support for Residential Care: Report of a joint central and local working party.*

Doty P (1988) 'Long Term Care in International Perspective', *Health Care Financing Review*, 1988 supplement.

Family Policy Studies Centre (1989) 'Family Care in Focus', *Family Policy Studies Bulletin*, 6, Winter 1989, London.

Field F (1992) *Making Labour into the Party of Work, Wealth and Opportunity.* Fabian Society, London.

Fries J F (1980) 'Ageing, Natural Death and the Compression of Morbidity', *New England Journal of Medicine*, 303: 130–135.

Fries J F (1989) 'Compression of Morbidity: Near or far?' *Millbank Memorial Fund Quarterly*, 67: 208–232.

Glendinning C, McLaughlin E (1993) *Paying for Care: Lessons from Europe.* Social Security Advisory Committee Research Paper No 5. HMSO.

Gordon C (1988) 'The Myth of Family Care?' *Ageing and Society*, 8: 287–320.

Green H (1988) *General Household Survey 1985: Informal carers.* HMSO.

Gruenberg E M (1977) 'The Failure of Success', *Millbank Memorial Fund Quarterly*, 55: 3–24

Grundy E (1987) 'Longitudinal Perspectives on the Living Arrangements of the Elderly', in M Jeffreys ed *Growing Old in the Twentieth Century.* Routledge, London.

Grundy E (1992) 'Socio-Demographic Change', in *The Health of Elderly People: An epidemiological overview*, Companion Papers to Volume 1, Department of Health. HMSO, London.

Grundy E, Harrop A (1992) 'Co-Residence Between Adult Children and their Elderly Parents in England and Wales', *Journal of Social Policy*, 21/3: 325–348.

Hamnett C (1992) *Inheritance in Britain: The disappearing billions.* Report commissioned by PPP Lifetime plc, Stratford-upon-Avon.

Hill J (1992) 'Does Britain Have a Welfare Generation?' *Oxford Review of Economic Policy*, 8/2, Summer 1992.

HMSO (1986) *Making a Reality of Community Care.* Report of the Audit Commission for England and Wales.

HMSO (1988a) *Community Care: Agenda for action.* Report to the Secretary of State for Social Services by Sir Roy Griffiths.

HMSO (1986b) *A Positive Choice.* Report of the Independent Review of Residential Care chaired by Gillian Wagner.

HMSO (1989) *Caring for People: Community care in the next decade and beyond.* Department of Health, Cmnd 849, London.

HMSO (1990a) *Community Care: Carers.* Fifth report of the House of Commons Social Services Committee, Session 1989–90, p vii.

HMSO (1990b) *Public Expenditure on the Social Services: A memorandum from the DHSS.* House of Commons Session 1989–90.

HMSO (1990c) *Community Care: Choice for service users.* Sixth report of the House of Commons Social Services Committee, Session 1989–90.

HMSO (1991) *The Financing of Private Residential and Nursing Home Fees.* Fourth report of the House of Commons Social Security Committee, Session 1990–91.

HMSO (1992a) *Family Spending.* Report on the 1991 Family Expenditure Survey.

HMSO (1992b) *Population Projections 1989-based,* OPCS Series PP2 No 17.

HMSO (1992c) *The Government's Expenditure Plans 1992–93 to 1994–95.* Department of Health and Office of Population Censuses and Surveys Department Report, Cmnd 1913.

HMSO (1993) *Caring for People: Information pack for the voluntary and private sectors*. Department of Health.

Johnson P (1992) *Income: Pensions, earnings and savings in the Third Age*. Carnegie Inquiry into the Third Age, Research Paper No. 2, Carnegie United Kingdom Trust, Dunfermline.

Johnstone C (1991) *Homecare: A major market opportunity*. Paper given at Laing & Buisson's 4th Annual Elderly Care Conference, March 1991. Laing & Buisson, London.

Kestenbaum A (1993a) *Taking Care in the Market*. Independent Living fund, Nottingham.

Kestenbaum A (1993b) *Cash for Care*. Independent Living Fund, Nottingham.

Kramer M (1980) 'The Rising Pandemic of Mental Disorders and Associated Chronic Diseases and Disabilities, *Acta Psychiatr Scand*, 62: 282–297.

Laing W (1991) *Empowering the Elderly: Direct consumer funding of care services*. IEA Health and Welfare Unit, London.

Laing & Buisson (1993a) *Care of Elderly People: Market survey 1992/3*. London.

Laing & Buisson (1993b) *Laing's Review of Private Healthcare 1993*. London.

Levit K, Lazenby H, Cowan C, Letsch S (1991) 'National Health Expenditures 1990', *Health Care Financing Review*, 13, Fall 1991, 29–54.

Martin J, Meltzer H, Elliot D (1988) *The Prevalence of Disability among Adults*. OPCS Surveys of Disability in Great Britain, Report 1, HMSO.

Martin J, White A (1988) *The Financial Circumstances of Disabled Adults Living in Private Households*. OPCS Surveys of Disability in Great Britain, Report 2, HMSO, London.

McLaughlin E (1992) *Paying for Care: A conceptual scheme*. Paper presented to the Social and Health Research Society, Belfast, May 1992.

Meredith B (1993) *The Community Care Handbook: The new system explained*. Age Concern England, London.

Morris J (1993) *Community Care or Independent Living*. Joseph Rowntree Foundation, York.

Nationwide Anglia Building Society (1992) Personal communication.

OECD (1988a) *Reforming Public Pensions*. Paris.

OECD (1988b) *Ageing Populations: The social policy implications: Demographic change and public policy*. Paris.

Oldman C (1991) *Paying for Care*. Joseph Rowntree Foundation, York.

OPCS (1992) *Carers in 1990*. OPCS Monitor SS/92/2. Office of Population Censuses and Surveys.

OPCS (1993) OPCS Monitor PP2 93/1. Office of Population Censuses and Surveys.

Parker G (1990) *With Due Care and Attention: A review of research on informal care*. Family Policy Studies Centre, London.

Parker G, Lawton D (1991) *Further Analysis of the 1985 General Household Survey Data on Informal Care. Report 3: Carers and services*. Social Policy Research Unit, University of York.

Pattie A, Heaton J (1990) *A Comparative Study of Dependency and Provision of Care for the Elderly in the State and Private Sectors in the York District*. Yorkshire Regional Health Authority.

RICA (1988) *Continuing Care Communities: Research carried out for the Joseph Rowntree Memorial Housing Trust*. Research Institute for Consumer Affairs, London.

Rivlin A, Weiner J (1988) 'Who Should Pay for Long-Term Care for the Elderly?' *Brookings Review*, Summer 1988, Washington.

Robine J M, Ritchie K (1991) 'Healthy Life Expectancy: Evaluation of global indicator of change in population health', *British Medical Journal*, 302: 457–460.

Robins A, Wittenberg R (1992) 'The Health of Elderly People: Economic aspects', in *The Health of Elderly People: An epidemiological overview*, Companion Papers to Volume 1, Department of Health. HMSO, London.

Sinclair I, Parker R, Leat D, Williams J (1990) *The Kaleidoscope of Care: A preview of research on welfare provision for elderly people*. HMSO, London.

Smyth M, Browne F (1992) *1990 General Household Survey*. OPCS Social Survey Division, HMSO, London.

Sullivan D F (1971) 'A Single Index of Mortality and Morbidity', *Health Services and Mental Health Administration (HSMHA) Health Reports*, 86: 347–354.

Thompson D (1986) 'Welfare and the Historians', in L Bonfield et al (ed) *The World We Have Gained*. Blackwell, Oxford.

Thompson D (1992) 'The Obligations of the Elderly', in P Johnson and J Falkingham (eds) *Ageing and Economic Welfare*. Sage, London.

Timaeus I (1986) 'Families and Households of the Elderly Population: Prospects for those approaching old age', *Ageing and Society*, 6: 271–293.

Townsend P (1962) *The Last Refuge*. Routledge & Kegan Paul, London.

Trebilcock D (1985) *Pensions and Related Benefits*. Study Course 100/041, Chartered Insurance Institute Tuition Service, London.

Twigg J (1992) *Carers: Research and practice*. HMSO, London.

Wade B, Sawyer L, Bell J (1981) *Different Care Provision for the Elderly*. Report to the DHSS by the Department of Social Administration, London School of Economics.

Wall R (1984) 'Residential Isolation of the Elderly: A comparison over time', *Ageing and Society*, 4: 483–503.

Weiner J (1992a) Unpublished paper prepared for the OECD meeting on care of frail elderly people, 2–4 November 1992.

Weiner J (1992b) Personal communication. The Brookings Institute, Washington DC.

Wicks M (1992) Hansard, 30 November, Vol 215 Col 64.

Wittenberg R (1989) *Prototype Insurance Policy for Long Term Care*. Government Economic Service Working Paper No. 105, Department of Health.

APPENDIX: STATE FUNDING SYSTEMS IN SELECTED OECD COUNTRIES

Canada

	Places	Means test for public finance			Is owner-occupied home counted as an asset?
		Individual's income	*Individual's assets*	*Family*	
Long-stay hospitals	20 000 approx	See Nursing homes below			
Nursing homes	130 000 approx	No income test. Access to nursing home care is universally available on a non-means-tested basis under the Canadian Health Act. Charges (co-payments) vary by province but are typically set at a flat rate of $750 per month for a shared room or $1,700 per month for a private room. This is intended to pay for the housing/board part of costs. The minimum pensioner income, by comparison, is about $900 per month. Both for-profit and not-for-profit nursing homes are eligible to receive state funding	No assets test	No family contribution	No

| Home care services | NA | Varies between provinces and within provinces – charges may be levied and may be means-tested. Proposals for reform of Canadian long-term care include increased emphasis on home care with improved and more equal access across provinces and fewer and lower fees | No assets test | No family contribution | No |

Eire

	Places	Means test for public finance			Is owner-occupied home counted as an asset?
		Individual's income	Individual's assets	Family	
Long-stay hospitals and state-run welfare homes	9 000	State will pay up to full cost of care – elderly individuals contribute according to means	Any assets over £8 000 have to be spent down before an individual is eligible for state financial support	No family contribution	No
Private and voluntary nursing homes	9 000	State will pay up to £51 per week for care in approved homes (total 3 000 beds) – individuals contribute according to means	Any assets over £8 000 have to be spent down before an individual is eligible for state financial support	No family contribution	No
DOMICILIARY CARE					
Community health services	NA	State pays for home nursing for Category 1 persons*	No assets test	No family contribution	No
Local authority social services	NA	–	–	–	–

* Category 1 persons are those who pass a means test indicating they are unable to pay for health care services out of their own resources and who receive a full eligibility medical card.

In Eire, people with a low income are classed as Category I by the National Health Service and are eligible for a 'medical card' entitling them to free medical services, including long-term care in *state institutions*. The great majority of elderly people qualify for a medical card.

In addition, the state is obliged to provide institutional assistance and to recover the cost according to ability to pay for those people without a full eligibility medical card.

Both Category I ('fully eligible') residents and those who are 'assisted' by the state can only receive something approaching the full cost of care (average £150–£180 per week – range £100–£300 per week) if they are placed in a state institution; there are about 9,000 such places in Eire.

State funding is only available for care in private and voluntary (often religious) establishments, under very restrictive conditions. There are 9,000 beds in private and voluntary nursing homes, but only about 3,000 of these are in establishments which are approved by the Minister of Health to receive public sector 'subventions'; no nursing homes have been added to the approved list since 1980.

Fully eligible and assisted people can receive public funds in these approved establishments, but only up to £51 per week (1992) and the balance has to be paid by their families, etc.

Shortages of state and approved private facilities have led to some public money finding its way into non-approved private facilities. Thus in the Eastern Health Board area (around Dublin), where shortages are greatest, state-funded individuals who are receiving respite care, or who are 'destined' for a state sector bed, may have their costs paid in full by the Health Board. Sometimes, even ordinary long-term care residents may have the whole of their weekly fees paid for by the Health Board (less the patient's contribution in the case of 'assisted' people).

The Health (Nursing Homes) Act 1990 has not yet been implemented, but when it is it will create more demands on the state. The Act allows a state subvention to be paid by the relevant Health Board, for a person who has been properly needs-assessed and means-tested, in any nursing home.

Apart from this Act, there has been little discussion of the financing of long-term care in Eire.

France

	Places	Means test for public finance			Is owner-occupied home counted as an asset?
		Individual's income	*Individual's assets*	*Family*	
Long-stay hospitals	60 000	Hotel costs (*hebergement*) only are means-tested, with residents liable to pay all of their income, except for pocket money, towards this element of cost. Care costs (*soins*) are not means-tested. Health insurance funds pay FF202.20 per day, paid direct to institution	Hotel costs only are means-tested. People must exhaust their assets before being eligible for state support for this element of cost. No asset test for the care element	A small contribution may be sought from children	Yes, for hotel costs
Care homes *with nursing care*	81 000	Hotel costs means-tested as above. Non-means-tested contribution to care costs from health insurance fund is FF124.90 per day	Assets must be exhausted for eligibility for state support for hotel costs. No asset test for the care element	A small contribution may be sought from children	Yes, for hotel costs
without nursing care	221 000	As above, but health insurance contribution is FF16.40 per day	As above	As above	As above
Other institutions for elderly people	217 000	Includes places in *logements-foyer*, similar to sheltered housing. There is no health insurance contribution and any state support is income-tested	Any state support is asset-tested	As above	As above

DOMICILIARY CARE

Community health services	NA	Non-means-tested right to medically prescribed nursing at home – up to 4 visits per day of up to 30 minutes each or up to 2 visits per day of up to 6 hours each	No assets test	No family contribution	No
Local authority social services	NA	Home help services are charged on sliding scale depending on income	No assets test	No family contribution	No

Private long-term care insurance was introduced by three insurance companies in France in the mid-1980s.

One of the companies introduced a comprehensive package of long-term care benefits but sales were poor and the product is no longer marketed. As in Germany (see below) poor sales were attributed to the high cost of the package and lack of awareness about the need for private provision. Insurance industry organisations are now looking afresh at the scope for private long-term care funding, with a view to introducing a more flexible range of products.

Germany

	Places	Means test for public finance			Is owner-occupied home counted as an asset?
		Individual's income	Individual's assets	Family	
Long-stay hospitals	Few	No income test. Only in Berlin do hospitals officially provide long-term care – though significant numbers of elderly people receive long-term care unofficially in hospitals in other parts of Germany. Average length of stay in German hospitals is unusually high	No assets test	No family contribution	No
CARE HOMES					
Public	103 000	Yes – strictly means-tested benefits are available from 'Social Help', the German equivalent of Income Support. Only care homes with an agreement with the public authorities are eligible to receive such state funds. Most private (for-profit) care homes do not have such an agreement	Yes – elderly people must spend down to DM4,500 to be eligible for state funding	Yes – sons, but not daughters must contribute a relatively modest sum to the cost of parents' care	Yes – and there is a bar on divestment up to 10 years previously
Voluntary	396 000				
Private	95 000				
DOMICILIARY CARE					
Community health services	NA	Nursing services of up to 2 hours per day are covered by sickness funds with no income test	No assets test	No family contribution	No

Local authority social services	NA	Access to personal care and domestic help is income-tested through Social Help	No assets test	No family contribution	No

Tensions arising from the severely means-tested system of state funding for long-term care led the German government to consider the inclusion of more generous long-term benefits through the sickness funds. Initially, because of financial considerations, this option was rejected and private funding alternatives were explored.

The German Life Assurance Association formed a committee with the remit of producing a model long-term care product to be offered for sale by the German life assurance industry. The product ( ) was introduced in 1985. It provided comprehensive benefits but was expensive and achieved few sales.

The disappointing results of the private sector initiative placed the issue back on the political agenda. The Liberal coalition partners argued for a mandatory private long-term care insurance scheme but the compromise eventually agreed with the Christian Democrat coalition partners was for a social insurance scheme. In 1992 the German legislature agreed in principle to create a new social insurance funding scheme by January 1996.

Public long-term care insurance will be added to the statutory health insurance fund which will pay non-means-tested benefits at a level which, in the case of nursing home care, is intended to cover the care element of nursing home charges. Nursing home benefit will be DM2,100 per month (or the 1986 equivalent). Current (1992) nursing home costs are between DM3,500 and DM4,000 per month. Means-testing under the proposed plan will apply to the hotel element of nursing home charges only.

It has been agreed that the cost of the proposed scheme (expected to amount to 1.7 per cent of payroll initially, as compared with 8–12 per cent of payroll for health care) will be paid half by employers' contributions and half by employees' contributions.

The outstanding issue is how employers are to be compensated. Employers' organisations claim they already have the highest payroll overheads in Europe. One proposal is to reduce initial employee entitlements to sick pay. Another is to reduce holiday entitlement. A problem is that any imposed solution will amount to a breach of the collective bargaining rights of trades unions, which are enshrined in law. The issue is controversial and has provoked industrial action in defence of existing sick pay and holiday entitlements.

The Netherlands

	Places	Means test for public finance			Is owner-occupied home counted as an asset?
		Individual's income	*Individual's assets*	*Family*	
Long-stay hospitals	Few	No income test	No assets test	No family contribution	No
Nursing homes	6 000	State funding for these medically orientated facilities is provided through the Exceptional Medical Expenses Scheme (AWBZ). Benefits are income-tested, but the personal contribution to charges is capped at 2,000 guilder per month	No assets test	No family contribution	No
Homes for the aged	130 000	State funding for these facilities is provided through social security grants to local authorities which apply an income test with no upper limit on personal contributions	Residents must exhaust their assets before being eligible for state funding	No family contribution	Yes
DOMICILIARY CARE					
Community health services	NA	AWBZ funds home nursing and day care in nursing homes on a non-means-tested basis with small personal charges	No assets test	No family contribution	No

Local authority social services	Professional home help services, meals on wheels and day centres are funded by local authorities with income-related charges. Non-professional 'Alpha' helpers who offer less intensive home help (eg for shopping) are employed directly by elderly people who can claim back part of the cost from the state if their income is low	NA	No assets test	No family contribution	No

The Exceptional Medical Expenses Scheme (AWBZ) came into force in 1967 to pay for a number of health care services not covered under ordinary health insurance, including nursing home care, day care in nursing homes and home nursing. Nursing home care was originally free under AWBZ, but a co-payment was introduced at the beginning of the 1980s. The co-payment is income-related with a cap of 2,000 guilder per month.

Under the Dekker reforms, which have yet to be implemented, it was proposed to bring medical care, all long-term care outside people's own homes, including both nursing homes and the much larger number of homes for the aged, home nursing, and professional home help within a revamped basic public health insurance scheme. The replacement of Liberals by Socialists in 1988 led to revisions. Some parts of the reforms have been implemented, others are still being discussed. Though the reforms ostensibly extend the range of the public health insurance scheme to cover more long-term care than before, their effect may be to *increase* the severity of means-testing. The income and assets means test with no upper limit on personal contributions, which is now applied to residents of homes for the aged, may be retained and applied to the currently less severely means-tested nursing home sector as well.

Sweden

	Places	Means test for public finance			Is owner-occupied home counted as an asset?
		Individual's income	*Individual's assets*	*Family*	
Long-stay hospitals	0	–	–	–	–
Nursing homes	51 000*	State funding for entry into a nursing home or a home for the aged is available subject to a charge which is income-related but varies according to municipality. Typical charges amount to 60–80 per cent of the individual's income	There is a limited assets test taking into account assets above the wealth tax threshold	No family contribution	Home is only taken into account if assets are above wealth tax threshold. It is limited to the tax value, not the higher open market value
Homes for the aged	45,000*				
DOMICILIARY CARE					
Community health services	NA	Domiciliary care is subject to income-related charges	No assets test	No family contribution	No
Local authority social services	NA	Domiciliary care is subject to income-related charges	No assets test	No family contribution	No

* There are also 40,000 flats for elderly people in congregate housing units (service flats), many of which have been converted from former nursing homes or homes for the aged.

164

Until recently, elderly people in Sweden were entitled to one year of long-term care outside their own homes free of any income-related charges. This was discontinued for reasons of economy.

United States

	Places	Means test for public finance			Is owner-occupied home counted as an asset?
		Individual's income	*Individual's assets*	*Family*	
Long-stay hospitals	0	–	–	–	–
CARE HOMES					
Skilled nursing	NA	No income test. Medicare, the federal health insurance scheme mainly for over-65s, pays non-means-tested benefits for skilled nursing care (covers rehabilitation only, not long-term care)	No assets test	No family contribution	No
Intermediate nursing	NA	No Medicare cover. Medicaid benefits are means-tested, leaving residents pocket money only	Elderly people must exhaust their assets before qualifying for Medicaid	No family contribution	Usually yes – the elderly person's home may be subject to a lien by Medicaid after death
Custodial care	NA				
DOMICILIARY CARE					
Home health care	NA	Limited non-means-tested Medicare home health care benefits	No assets test	No family contribution	No
Local authority social services	NA	Varies widely by state – services generally subject to charges	No assets test	No family contribution	No

Buchanan et al (1991) give the following data on sources of funding for nursing home care in the United States in 1989:

- $54.5 billion was spent on nursing home care, 8.4 per cent of total national health expenditure.
- $28 billion (51.3 per cent) came from private payments.
- $22.1 billion (40.6 per cent) came from the state welfare programme, Medicaid.
- Less than 3 per cent came from private health insurance together with the federal health insurance programme, Medicare.

Medicare provides a non-means-tested nursing home benefit for 'participating skilled nursing homes'. But care has to be geared to rehabilitation in order to qualify, average length of stay is only a month, and half of the skilled nursing homes do not participate in the programme. Medicare home health care is similarly restricted. Most elderly people in institutions are in 'custodial care' facilities which are not eligible for Medicare funding. The only state funding available for 'custodial care' residents is means-tested Medicaid.

The USA has the most highly developed private long-term care insurance sector in the world, but long-term care insurance still accounts for only 1 per cent of nursing home revenues.

There have been a number of proposals for reform of the severely means-tested system of public funding for long-term care, and a number of state initiatives aimed at reducing the severity of the means test and introducing private funding products which complement welfare entitlements.

With the election of Bill Clinton as President, a fundamental review of health care financing is to take place, which will include a review of long-term care financing.

ABOUT AGE CONCERN

Financing Long-Term Care is one of a wide range of publications produced by Age Concern England – National Council on Ageing. In addition, Age Concern is actively engaged in training, information provision, research and campaigning for older people and those who work with them. It is a registered charity dependent on public support for the continuation of its work.

Age Concern England links closely with Age Concern centres in Scotland, Wales and Northern Ireland to form a network of over 1,400 independent local UK groups. These groups, with the invaluable help of an estimated 250,000 volunteers, aim to improve the quality of life for older people and develop services appropriate to local needs and resources. These include advice and information, day care, visiting services, transport schemes, clubs, and specialist facilities for physically and mentally frail older people.

Age Concern England
1268 London Road
London SW16 4ER
Tel: 081-679 8000

Age Concern Wales
4th Floor
1 Cathedral Road
Cardiff CF1 9SD
Tel: 0222 371566

Age Concern Scotland
54a Fountainbridge
Edinburgh EH3 9PT
Tel: 031-228 5656

Age Concern Northern Ireland
3 Lower Crescent
Belfast BT7 1NR
Tel: 0232 245729

PUBLICATIONS FROM ◆A◆C◆E◆ BOOKS

A wide range of titles is published by Age Concern England under the ACE Books imprint.

■ Policy

Age: The unrecognised discrimination
Edited by Evelyn McEwen
Comprising a series of discursive essays by leading specialists on evidence of age discrimination in British society today, including the fields of employment, health care, leisure and the voluntary sector, this book is an important contribution to the growing debate.
£9.95   0–86242–094–6

The Coming of Age in Europe: Older people in the European Community
Written thematically, this set of eight essays provides a comparative study of social and welfare provision for older people across the countries of the EC and has been designed to act as a first point of reference on this important subject.
£12.95   0–86242–114–4

The Law and Vulnerable Elderly People
Edited by Sally Greengross
This report raises fundamental questions about the way society views and treats older people. The proposals put forward seek to enhance the self-determination and autonomy of vulnerable old people while

ensuring that those who are physically or mentally frail are better protected in the future.

£6.50   0–86242–050–4

The Living Will
Consent to treatment at the end of life: A Working Party Report
A report analysing the potential role of advance directives and in particular the 'living will'.
Co-published with Edward Arnold.

£6.99   0–34049–142–6

Uniting Generations: Studies in conflict and co-operation
Edited by David Hobman
This book examines one of the major social questions of the next decade. A number of distinguished experts explore such issues as: the rationing of housing, health and social care, the changing pattern of family dynamics and social values. Examples of inter-generational collaboration are reviewed, including mentoring.

£14.95   0–86242–125–X

To order books, please send a cheque or money order, payable to Age Concern England, to the address below. Postage and packing are free. Credit card orders may be made on 081-679 8000.

ACE Books (DEPT F)
Age Concern England
PO Box 9
London SW16 4EX

CONTINUING CARE PUBLICATIONS

Left Behind?
Continuing care for elderly people in NHS hospitals – A review of
Health Advisory Service reports
June 1990   8 pp   £1.00

Under Sentence
Continuing care units for older people within the National Health
Service – A discussion paper
December 1990   20 pp   £2.00

Dis-continuing Care
Report of a survey of district health authority plans for continuing
care of elderly people
June 1991   20 pp   £2.00

Home Help and Care
Rights, charging and reality
August 1992   28 pp   £2.50

For further information, or to order Continuing Care publications,
write to:

Donna Pearce
Age Concern England
1268 London Road
London SW16 4ER

INFORMATION FACTSHEETS

Age Concern England produces over 30 factsheets on a variety of subjects. Among these the following titles may be of interest to readers of this book:

Factsheet 6 *Finding Help at Home*

Factsheet 10 *Local Authority Charging Procedures for Residential and Nursing Home Care*

Factsheet 11 *Preserved Entitlement to Income Support for Residential and Nursing Homes*

Factsheet 29 *Finding Residential and Nursing Home Accommodation*

TO ORDER FACTSHEETS

Single copies are available free on receipt of a 9" x 6" sae. If you require a selection of factsheets or multiple copies totalling more than five, charges will be given on request.

A complete set of factsheets is available in a ring binder at the current cost of £34, which includes the first year's subscription. The current cost for annual subscription for subsequent years is £14. There are different rates of subscription for people living abroad.

Factsheets are revised and updated throughout the year and membership of the subscription service will ensure that your information is always current.

For further information, or to order factsheets, write to:

Information and Policy Department
Age Concern England
1268 London Road
London SW16 4ER

INDEX